GOING TO THE DOCTOR

Sheila Hollins,
Jane Bernal and Matthew Gregory

illustrated by Beth Webb

Books Beyond Words

St George's Mental Health Library

First published in Great Britain 1996.

Text copyright Sheila Hollins 1996.

Illustration copyright Sheila Hollins & Beth Webb 1996.

No part of this book may be reproduced in any form,
or by any means without the prior permission
in writing of the publisher.

ISBN 1874439 13 3

British Library Cataloguing-in-Publication Data.
A catalogue record for this book is available
from the British Library.

Typeset, printed and bound in Great Britain
by Acanthus Press Limited, Wellington, Somerset TA21 8ST.

Further information about the Books Beyond Words series
can be obtained from:

The Department of Psychiatry of Disability,
St. George's Hospital Medical School,
Cranmer Terrace, London SW17 ORE
Tel: 0181 725 5501   Fax: 0181 672 1070

Acknowledgements

We would like to thank our Editorial Advisers, Veronica Donaghy, Nigel Hollins and Lloyd Page, for helping us think of ideas for this book and telling us what was needed in the pictures.

Many people gave their time most generously, particularly Dr Bernadette Grimmet, Dr Ruth Ryan, Dr Andrew Flynn, Ingrid Edmunds, Jackie Rodgers, Julia Gale, Jenny Pearson, John Turnbull, Freda Macey and Dorothea Duncan. Thanks are also due to People First, Haywards Heath Health Group, the staff and clients in Wandsworth Community Health Trust and the Roehampton Community Team for People with Learning Disabilities, and staff and patients in the Phlebotomy Department, St. George's Hospital. Also the staff and patients of Wellington Medical Centre, Somerset.

Finally, *Going to the Doctor* would not have been possible without a generous grant from the Department of Health.

Contents

This book begins with two patients arriving at the health centre and then illustrates six possible scenarios which may occur during a visit to the surgery or health centre.

The Scenarios 1, 2 & 3 show Jim Lane and Scenarios 4, 5 & 6 depict Ann Smith.

Always start with the introductory pictures showing patients arriving at the health centre or surgery.

Then choose the scenario which is most similar to the procedure or intervention which is planned. Each scenario includes pictures to enable the doctor or nurse to obtain the patient's consent.

Further advice on how to use this resource is provided in the guides after the pictures.

	page	divider colour
Introduction: Jim Lane and Ann Smith arrive at the Health Centre	1	blue
Scenario		
1. Something odd happens: Jim Lane has his blood pressure checked	8	purple
2. Something embarrassing happens: the doctor examines his tummy	15	orange
3. Something hurts: Jim Lane has an injection	23	yellow-orange
4. Something makes me better: Ann Smith has her ears syringed	30	yellow
5. Something pricks: Ann Smith has a blood test	40	green
6. Something to make me better: The doctor gives Ann Smith a prescription	49	cyan
Suggested text for each scenario	57	lilac
Guide for supporters/informants	64	lilac
Medical words explained	66	lilac
Guide for GPs and the Primary Care Team	68	lilac

Mr Lane and Miss Smith arrive at the Health Centre

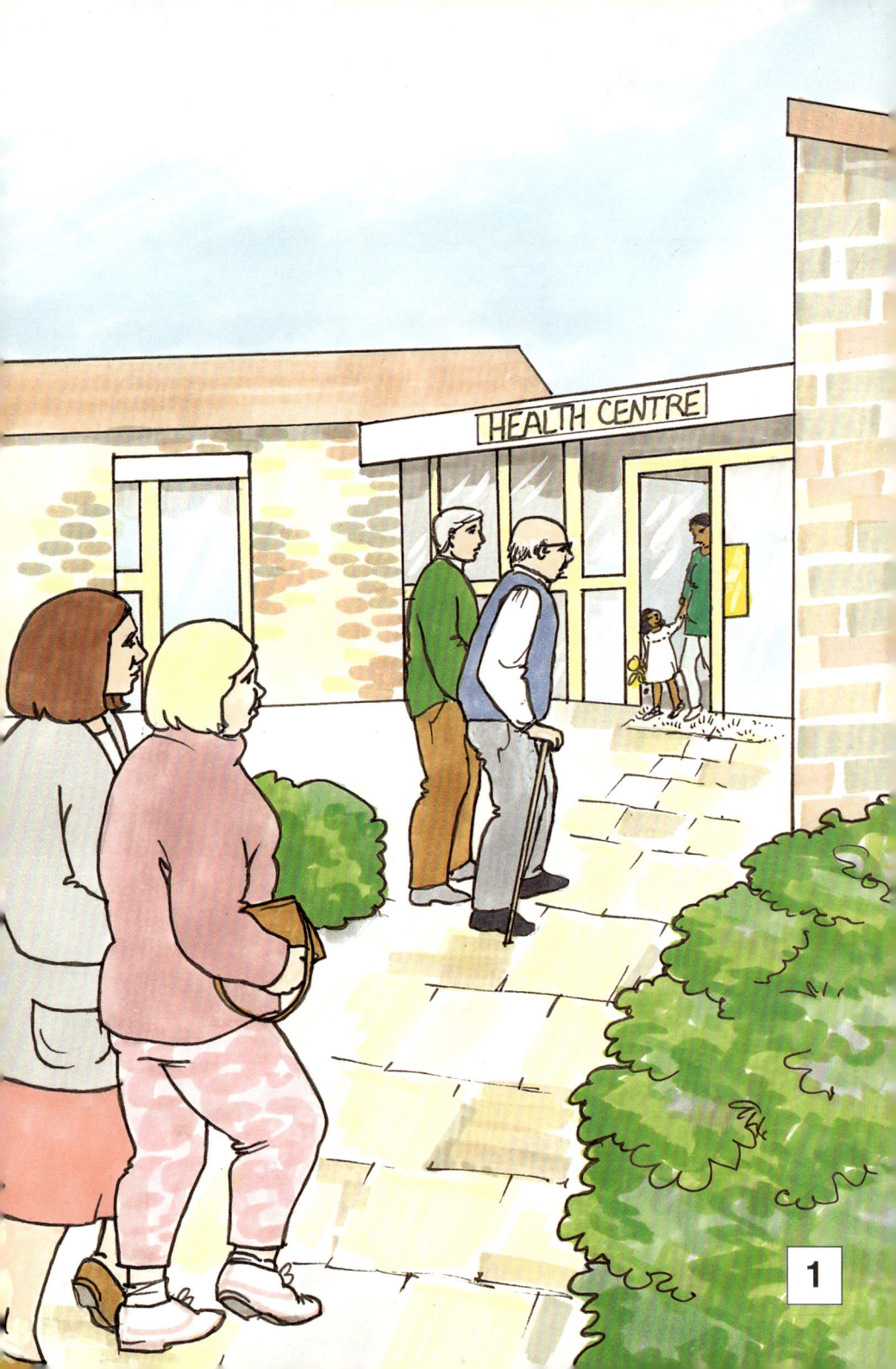

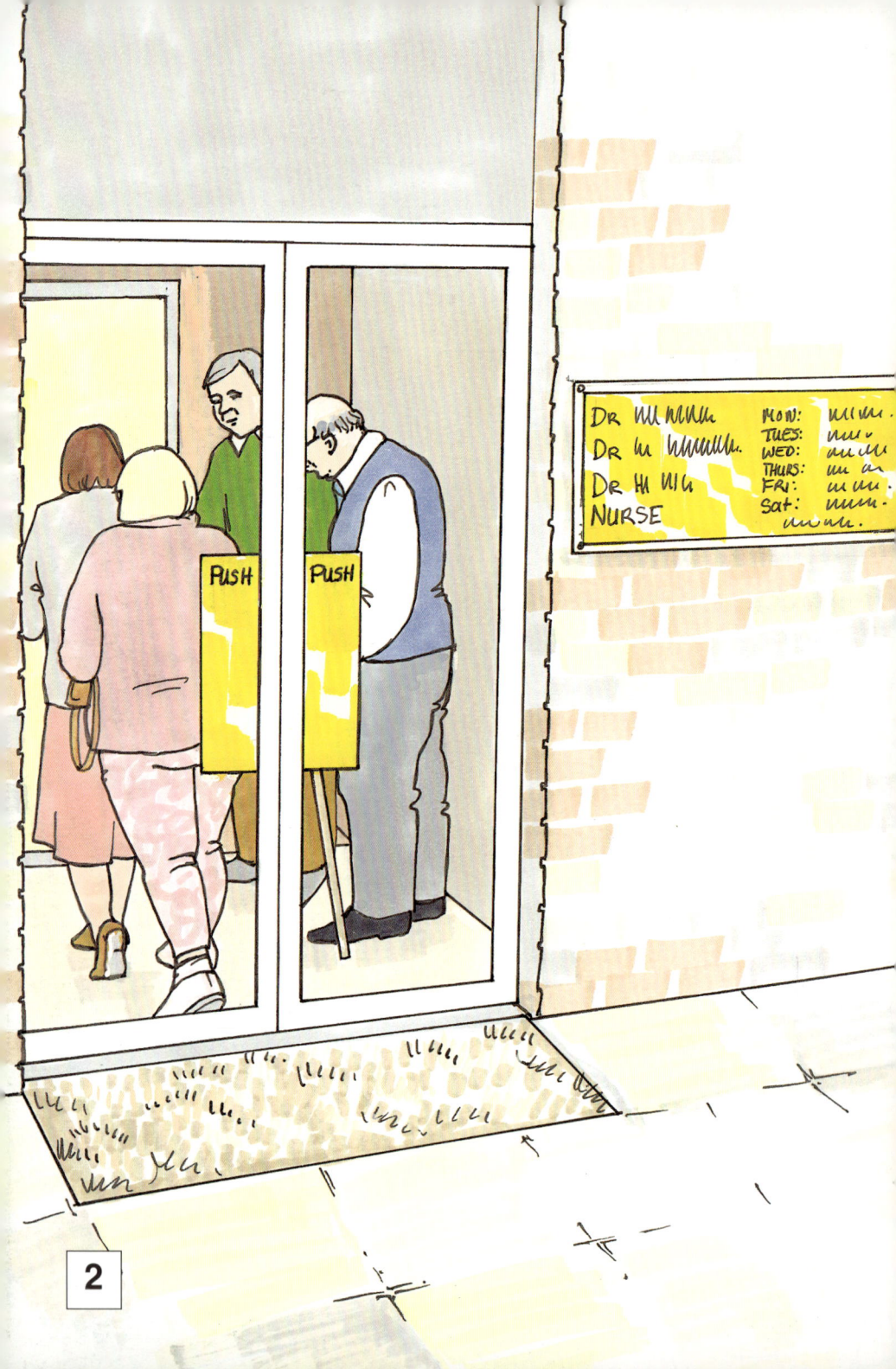

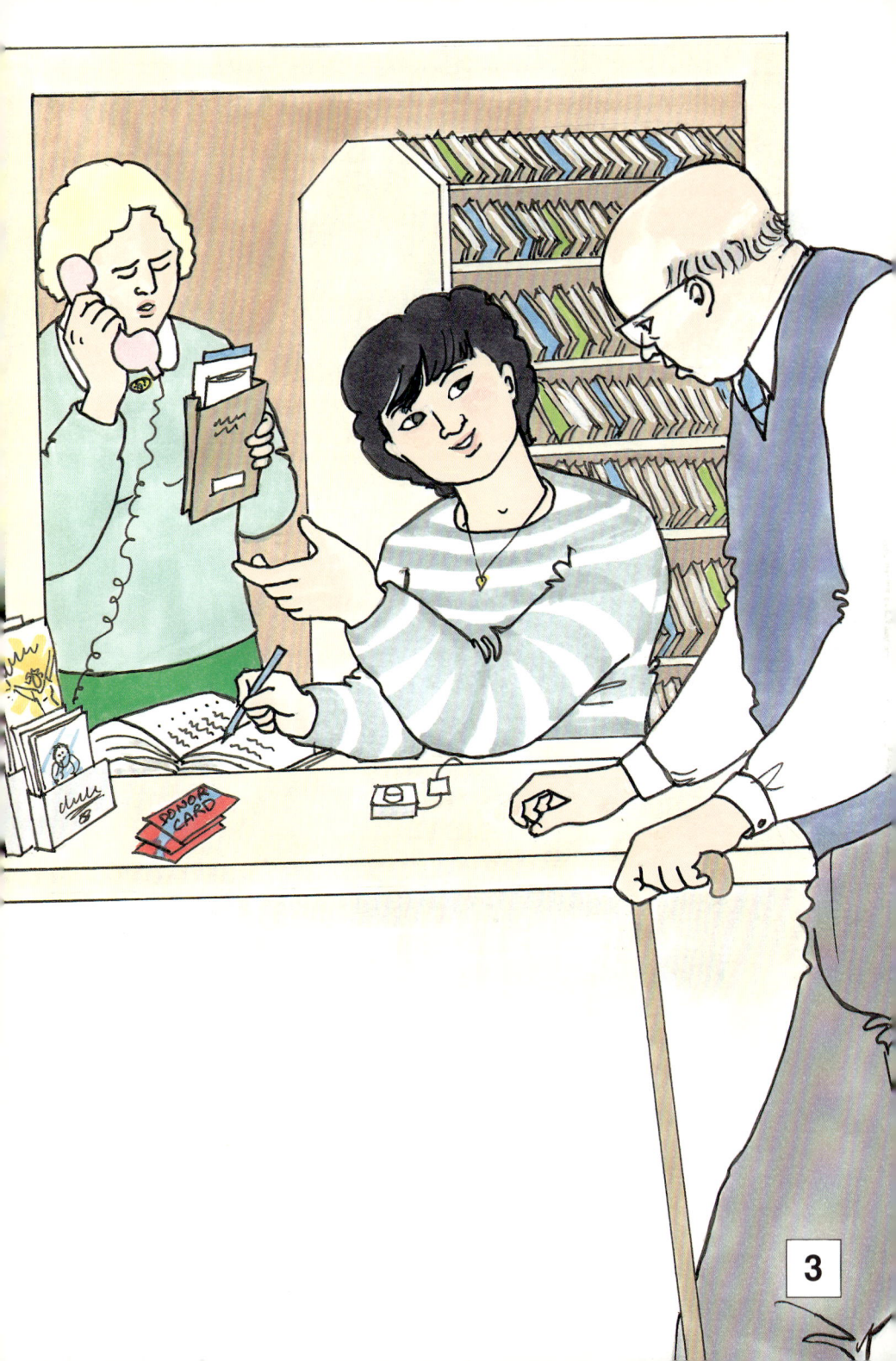

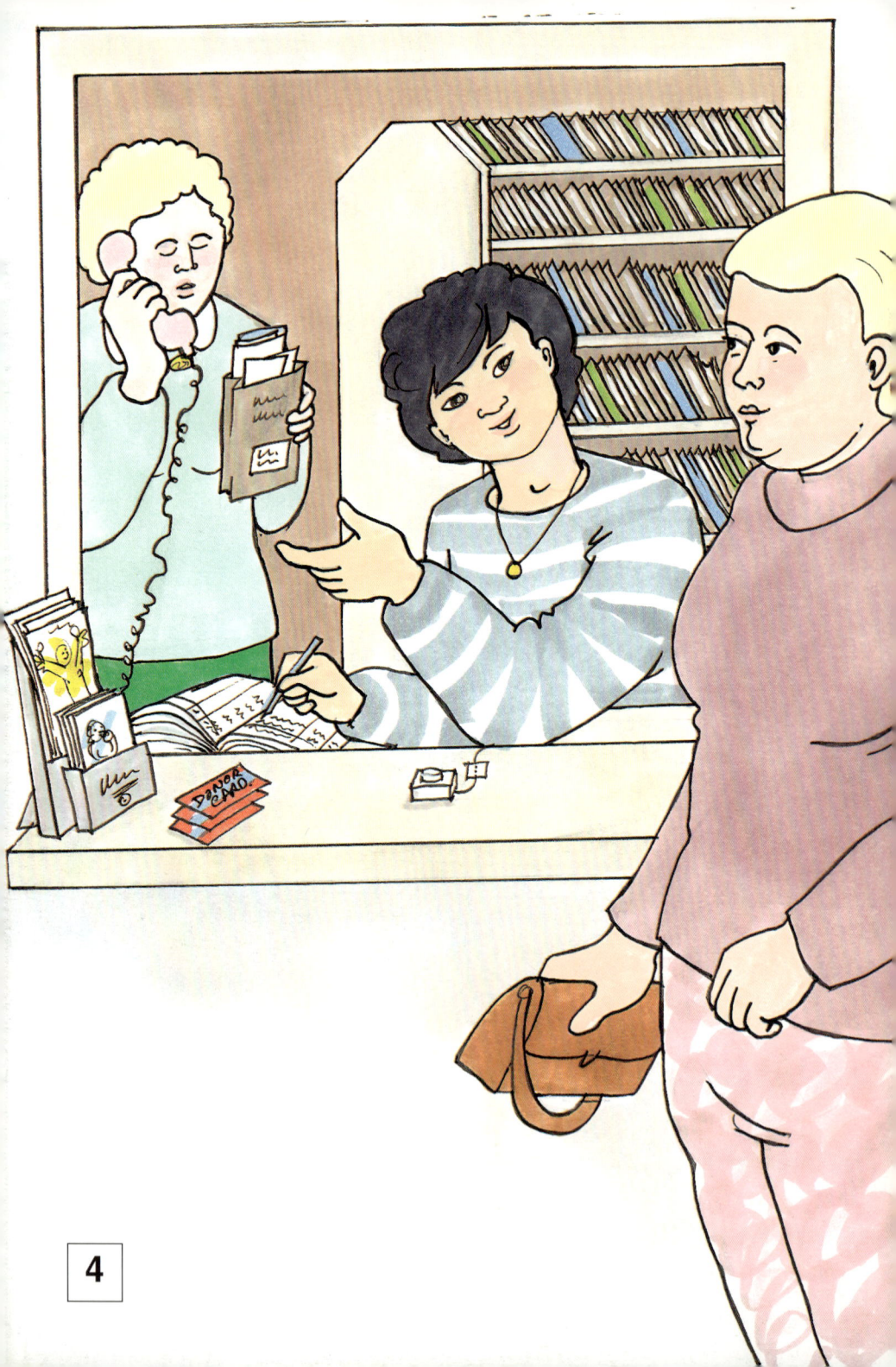

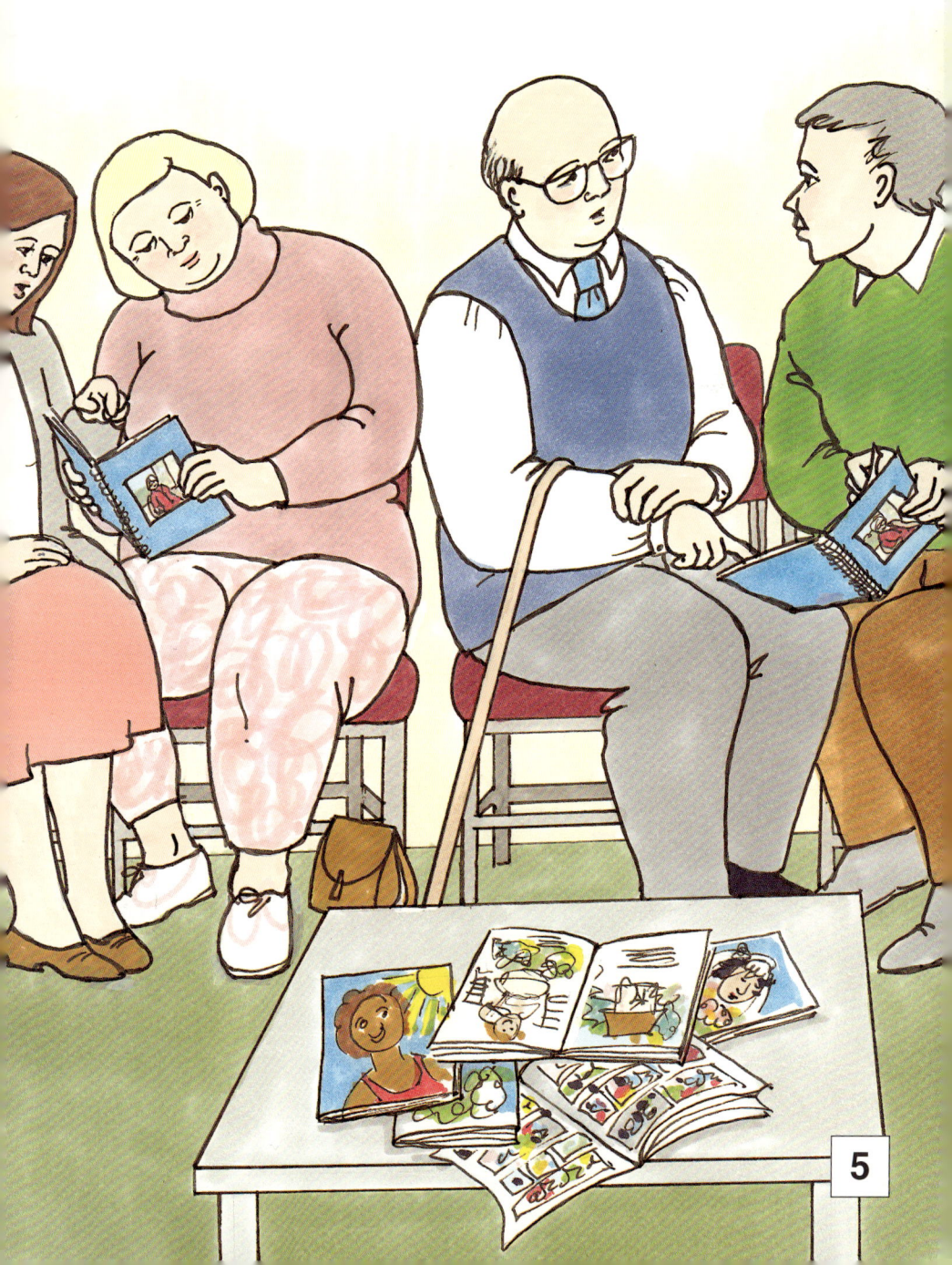

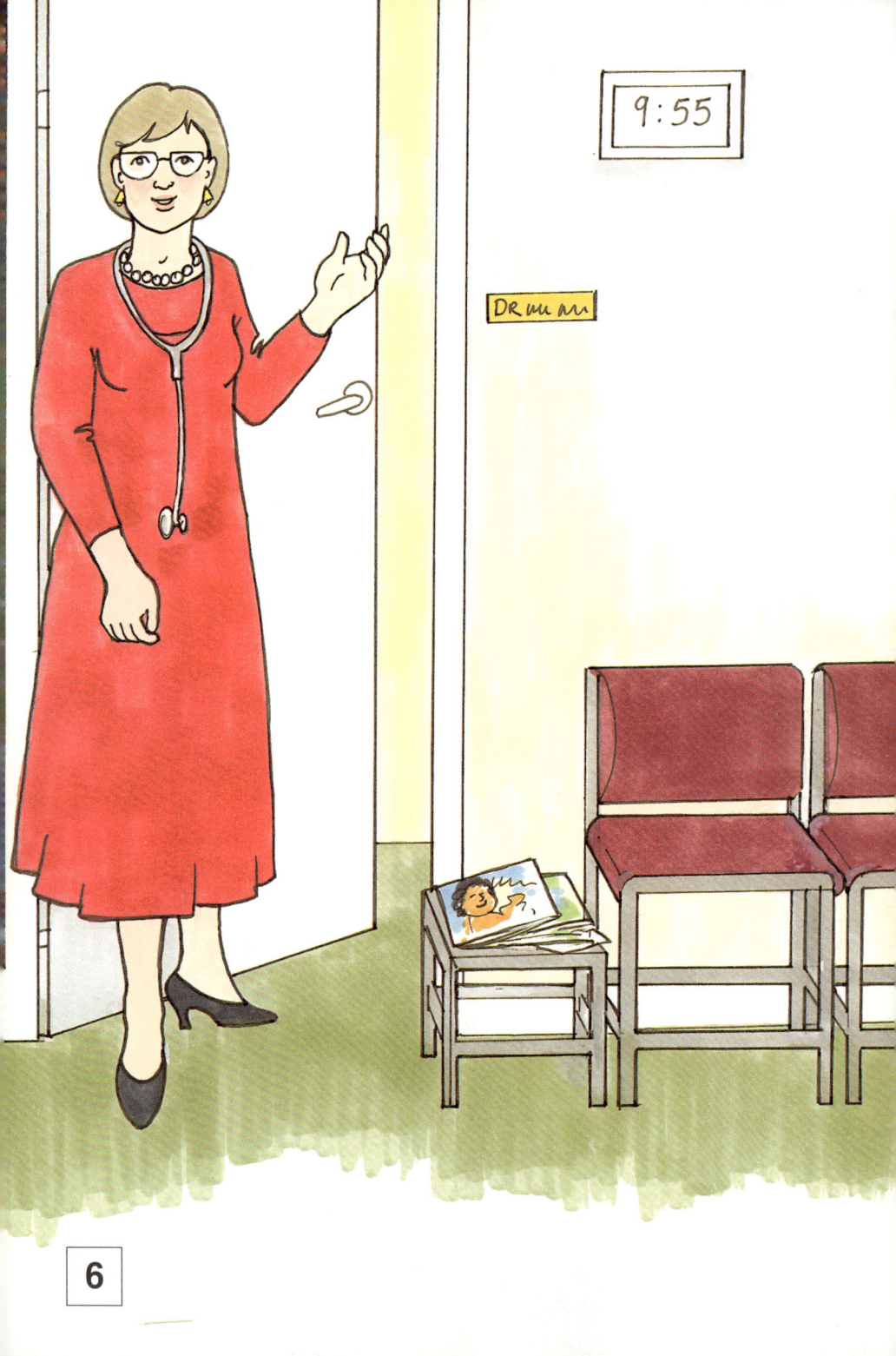

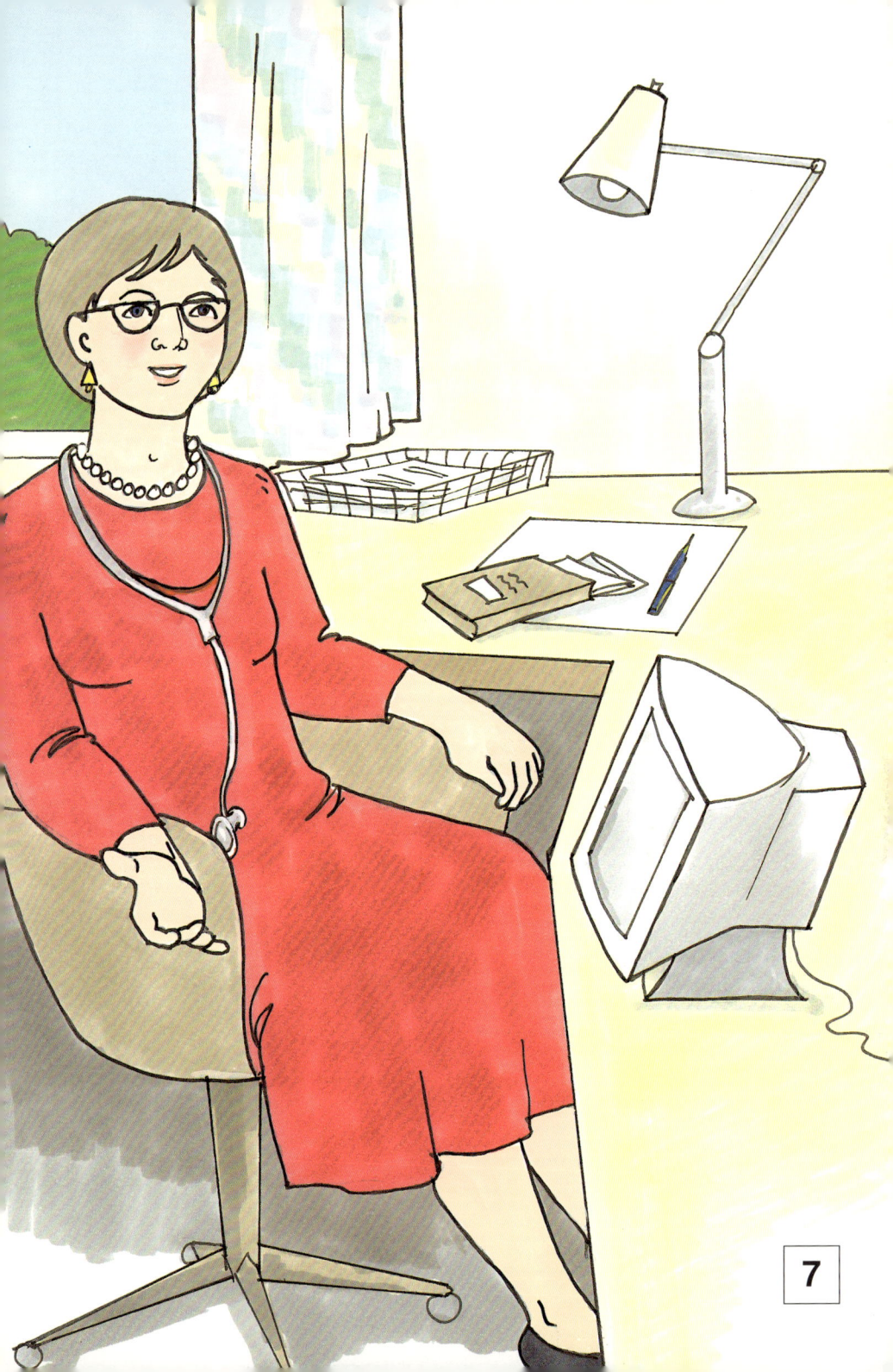

Now turn to the correct procedure — see the labelled dividers or the Contents Page

1: Blood Pressure

'Something odd happens'

Mr Lane has his blood pressure checked

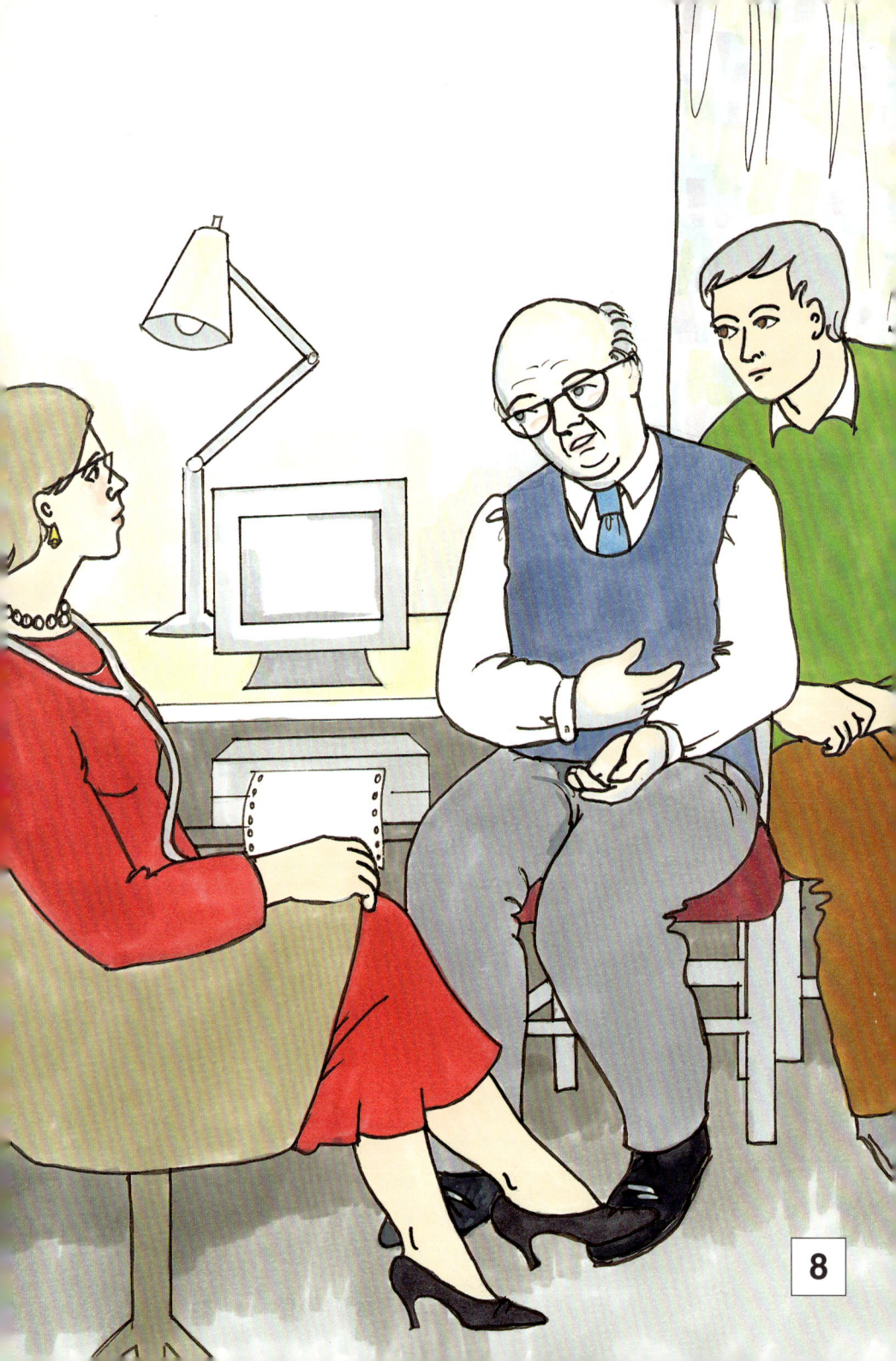

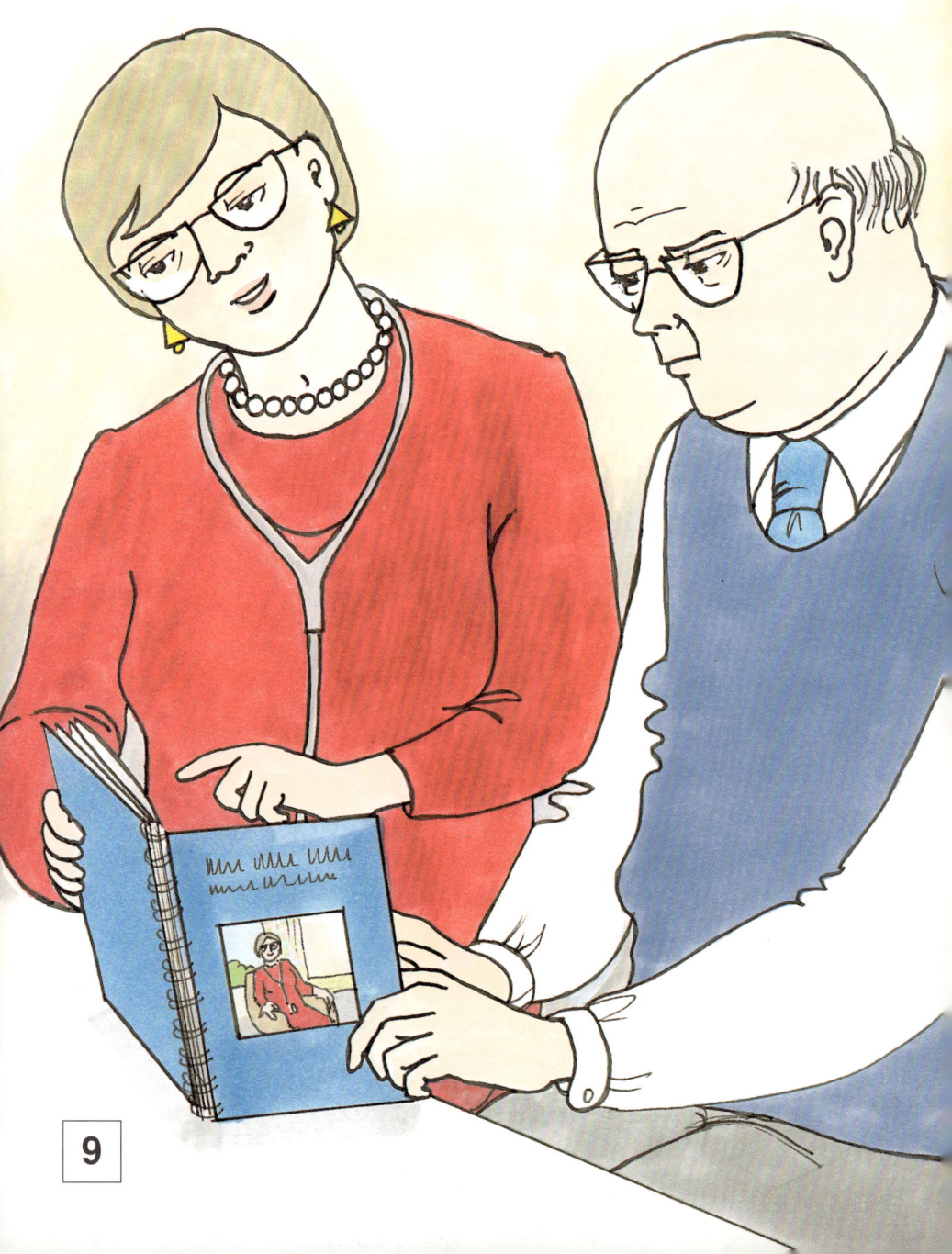

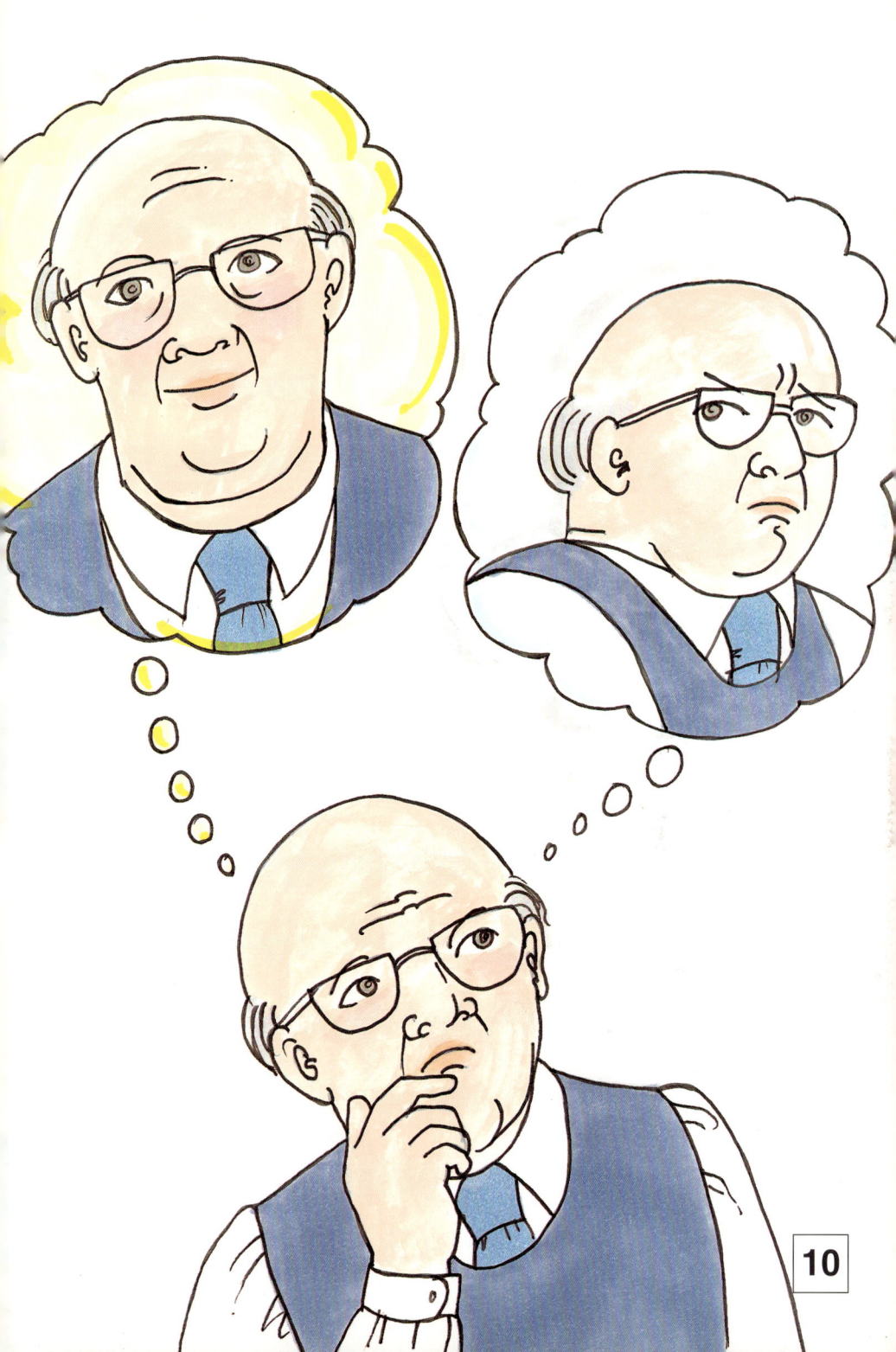

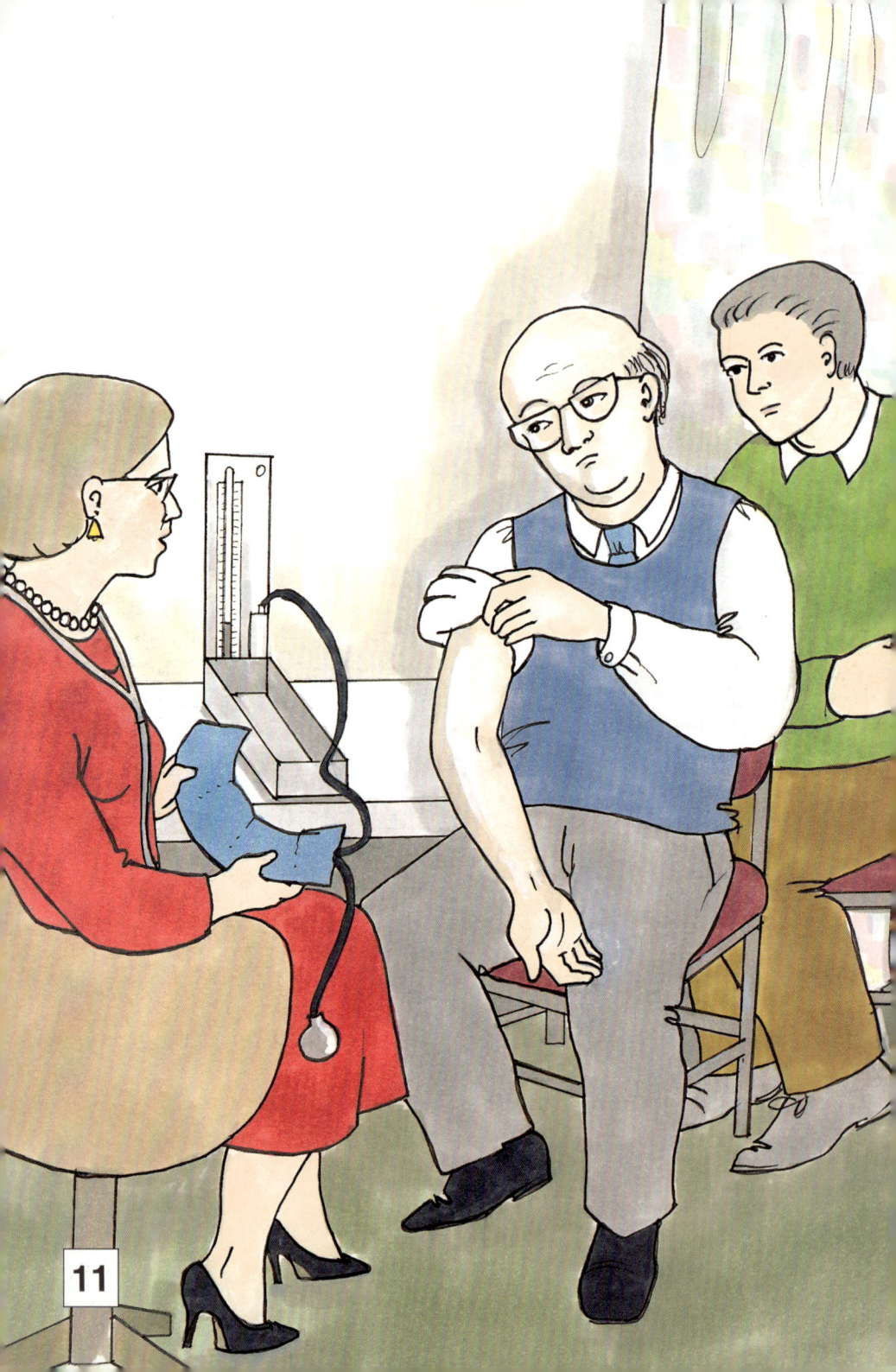

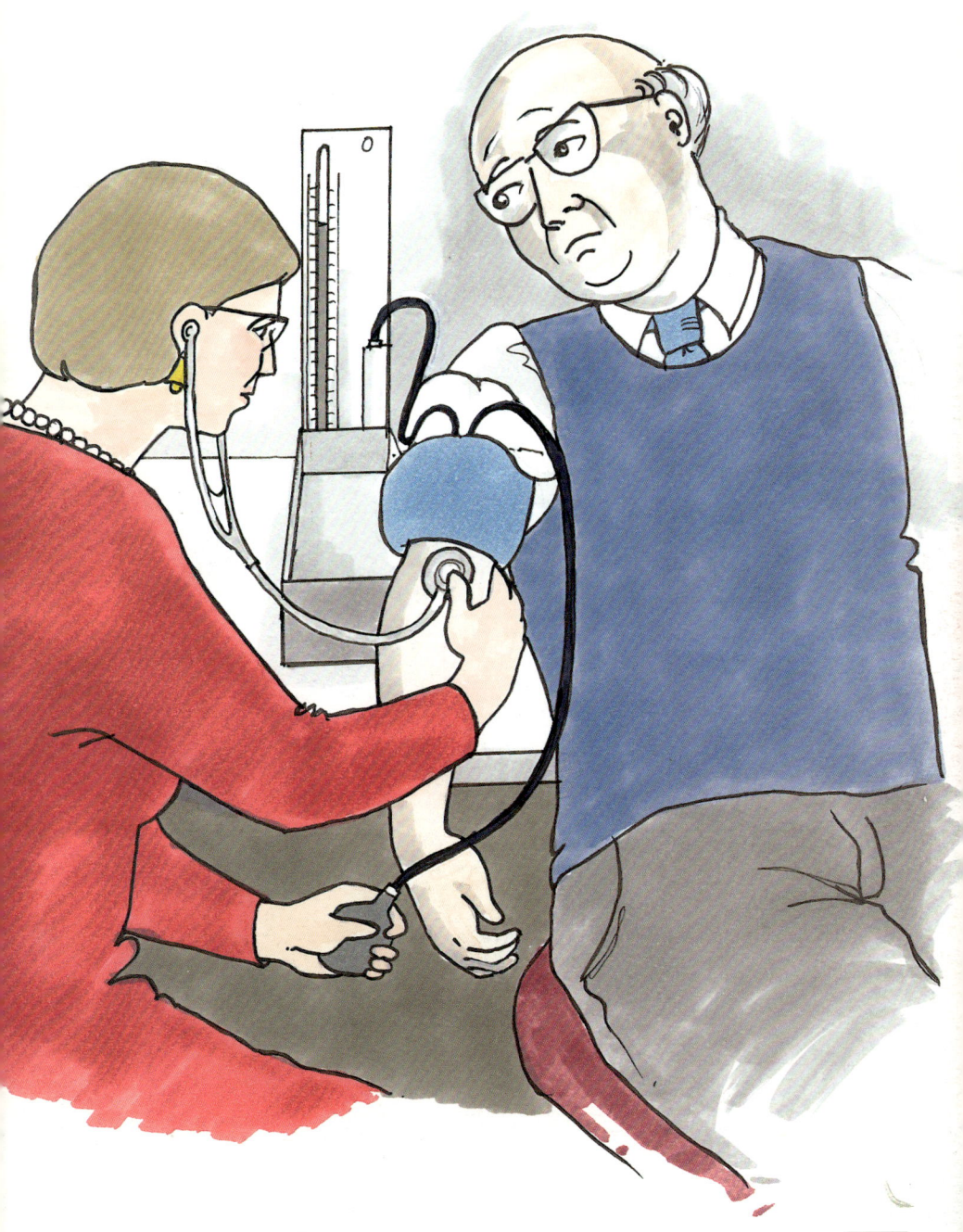

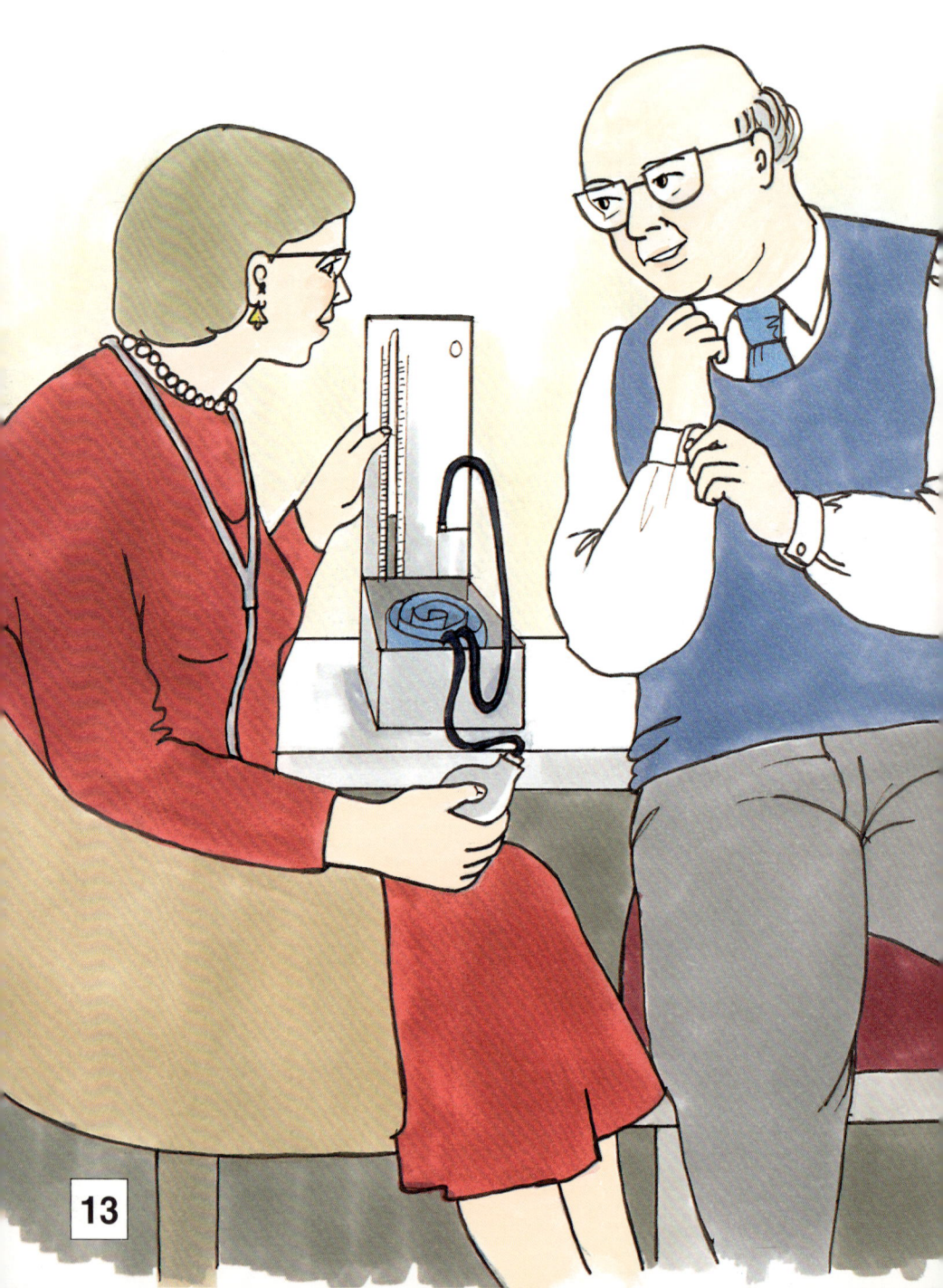

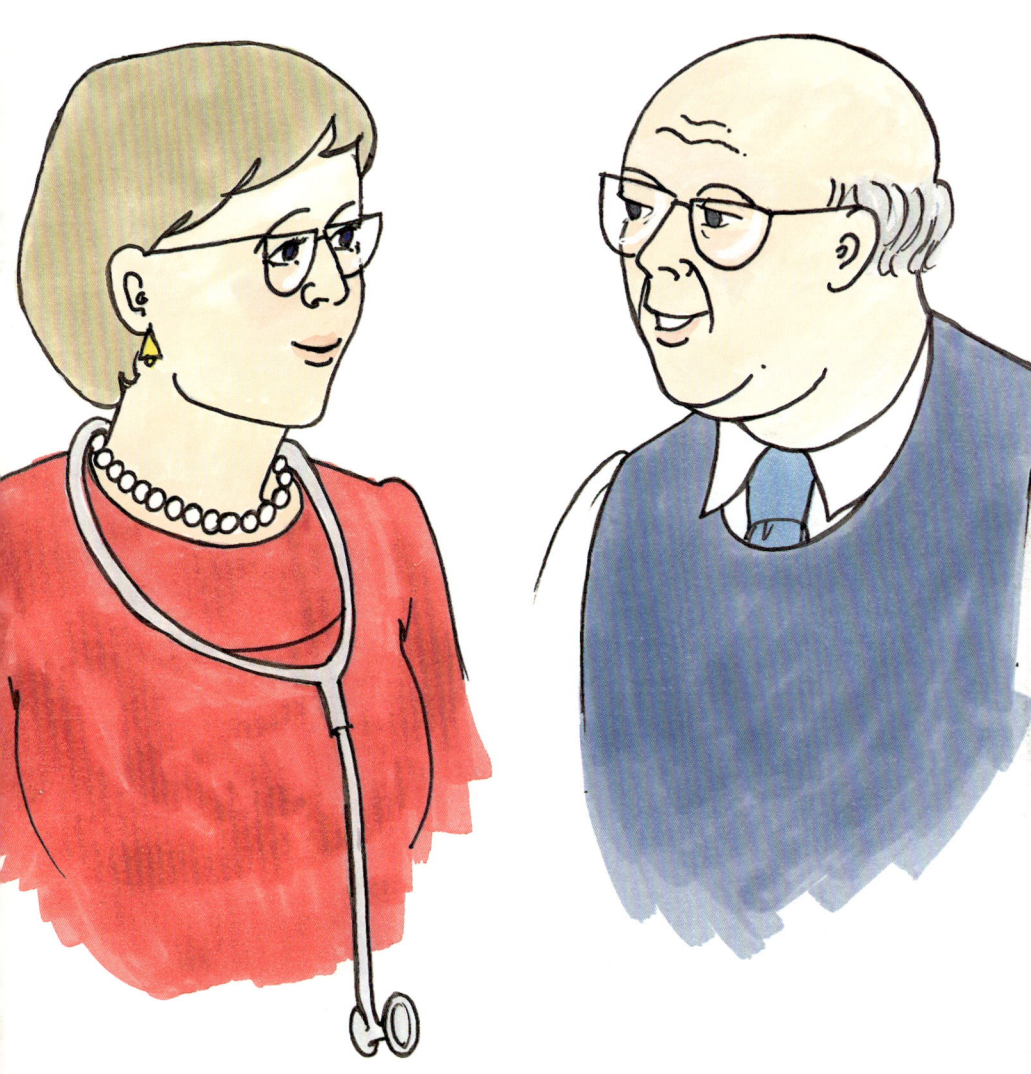

'Something embarrassing happens'

The doctor examines Mr Lane's tummy

2: Being Examined

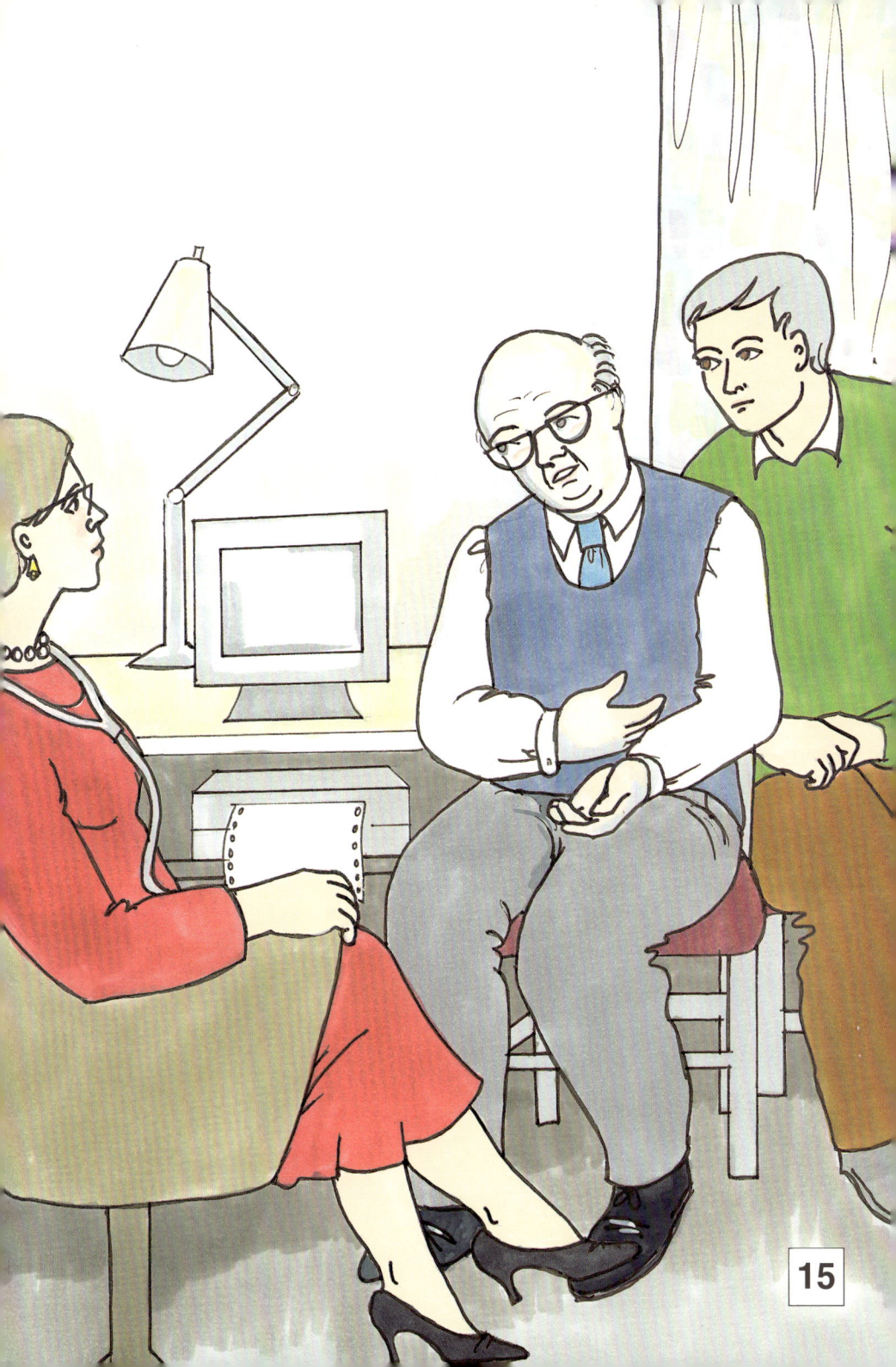

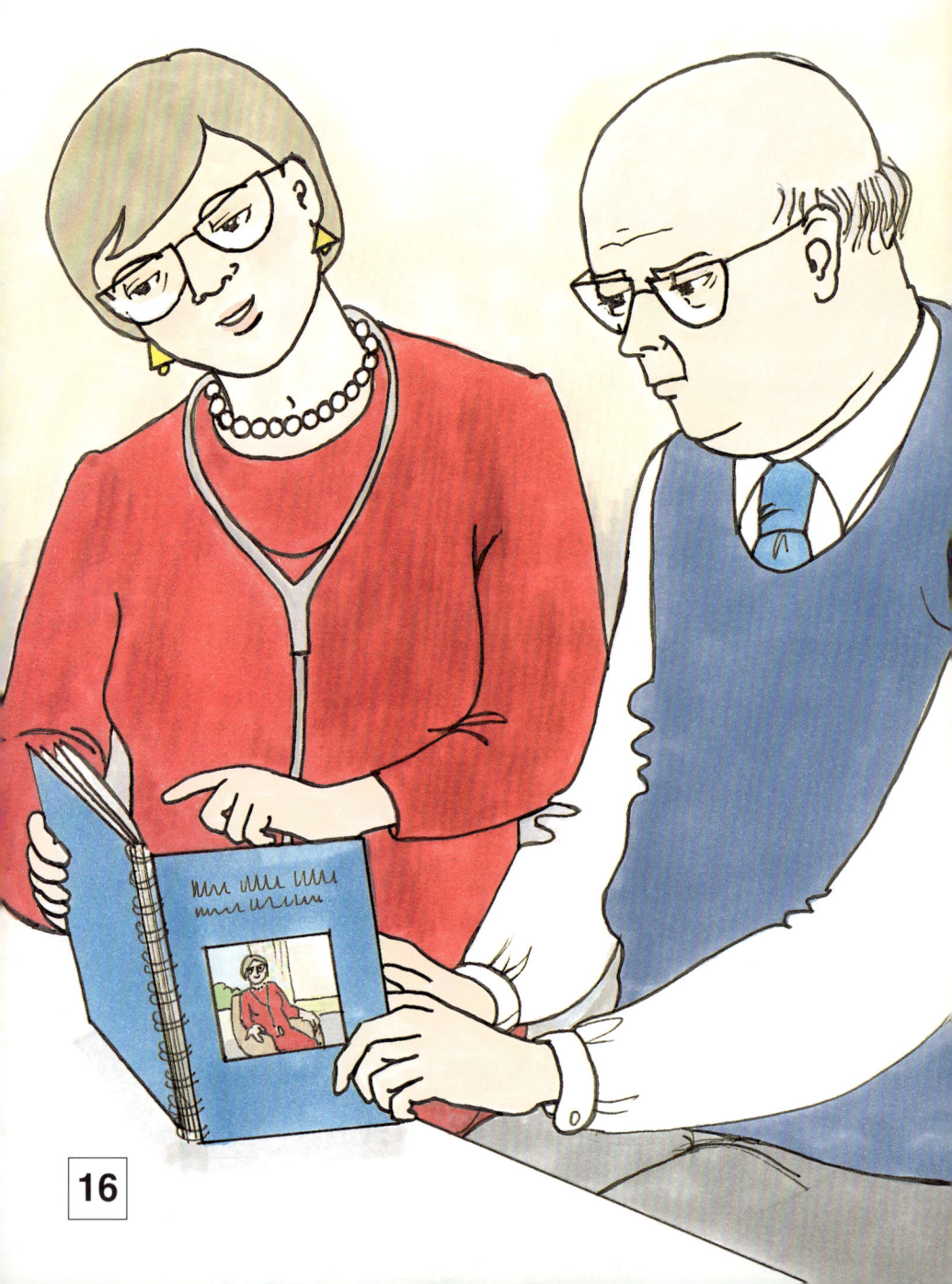

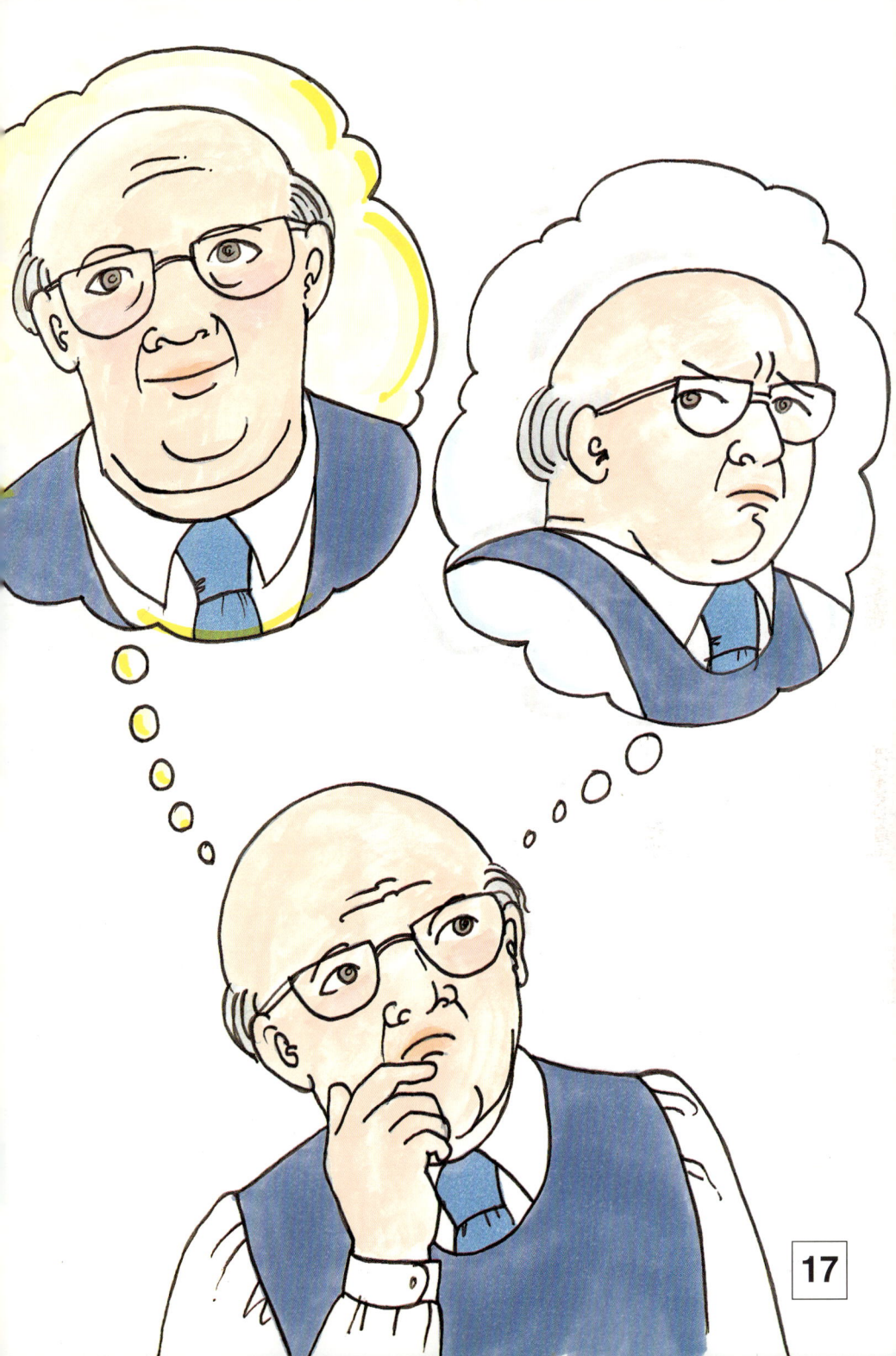

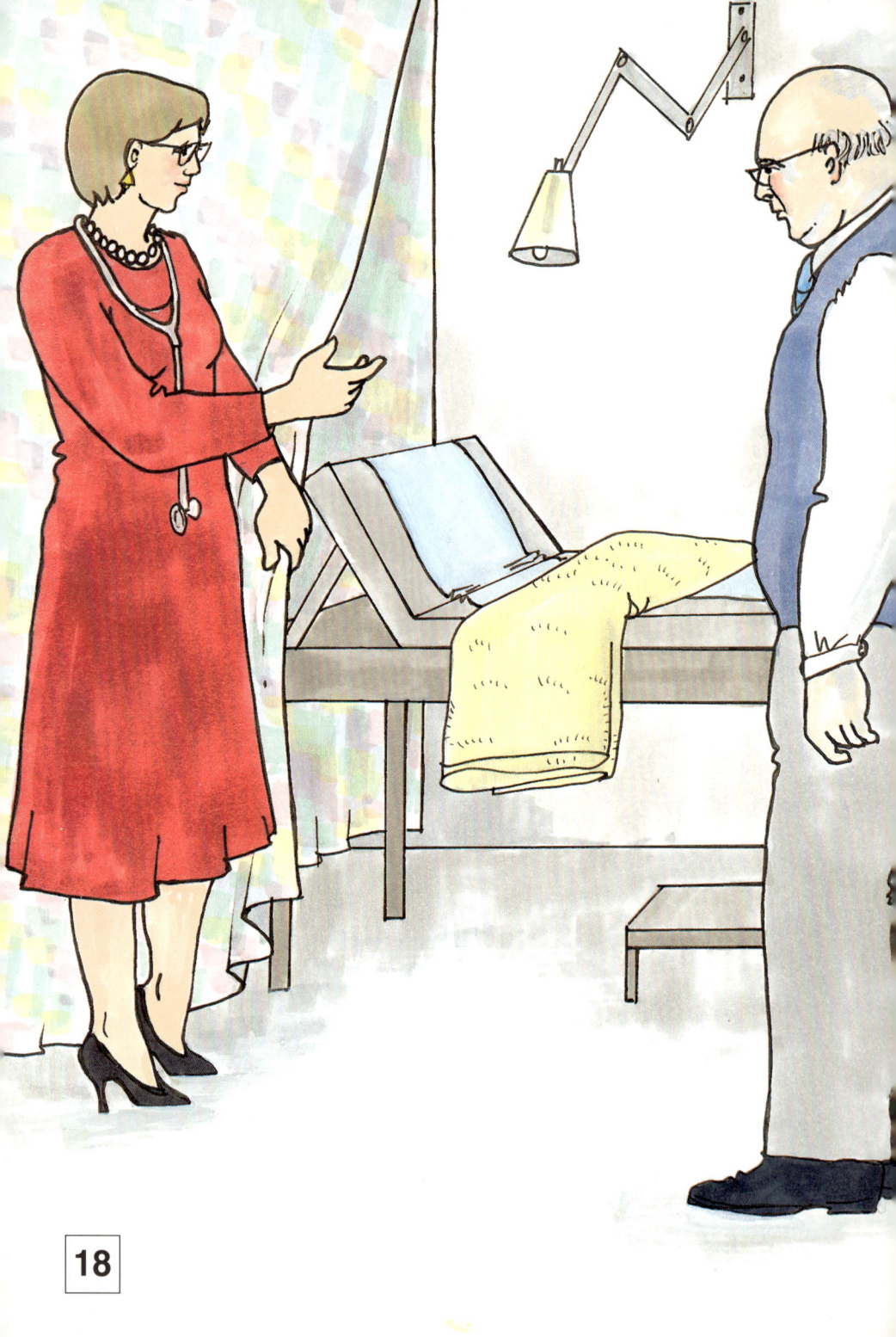

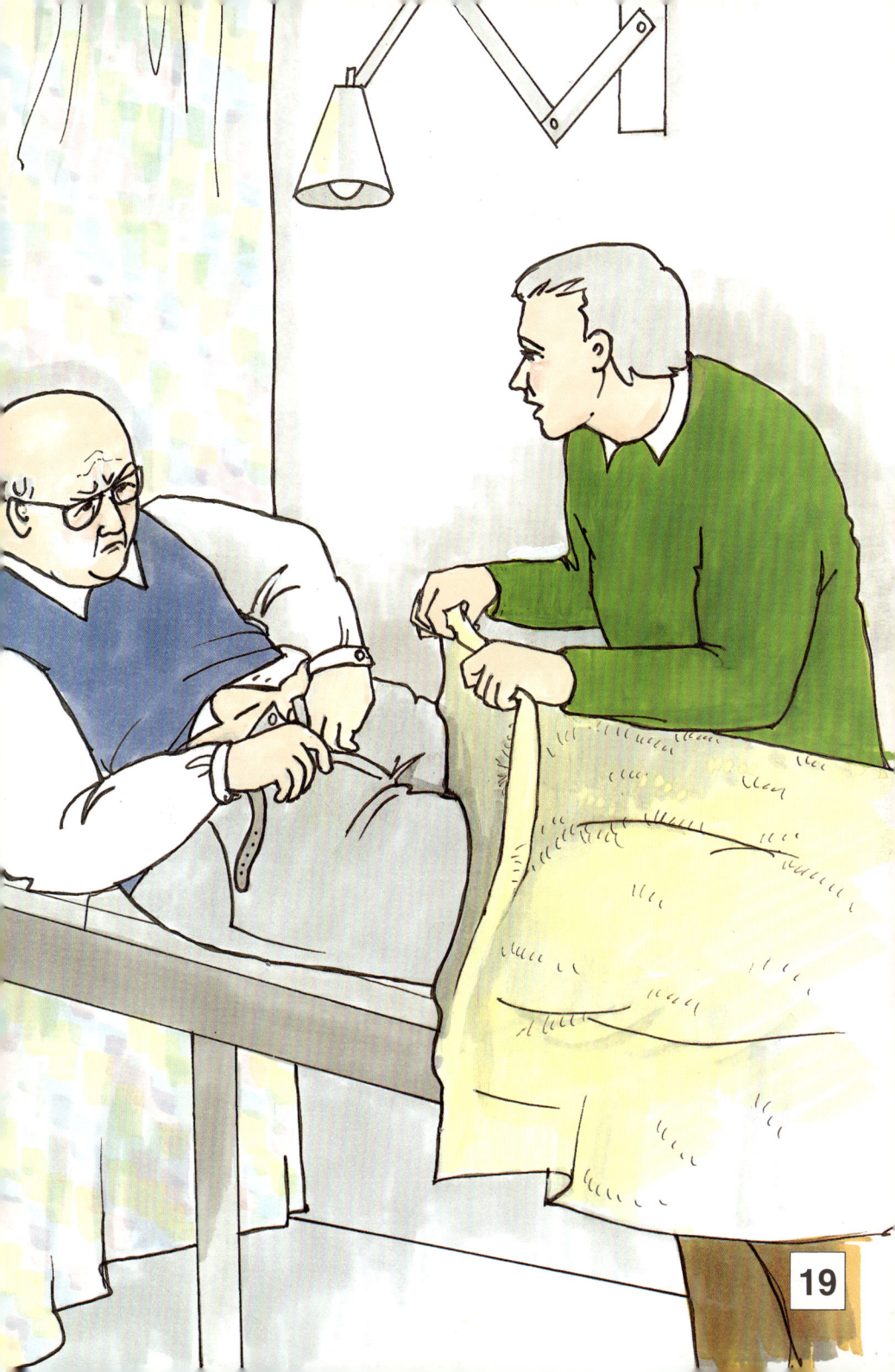

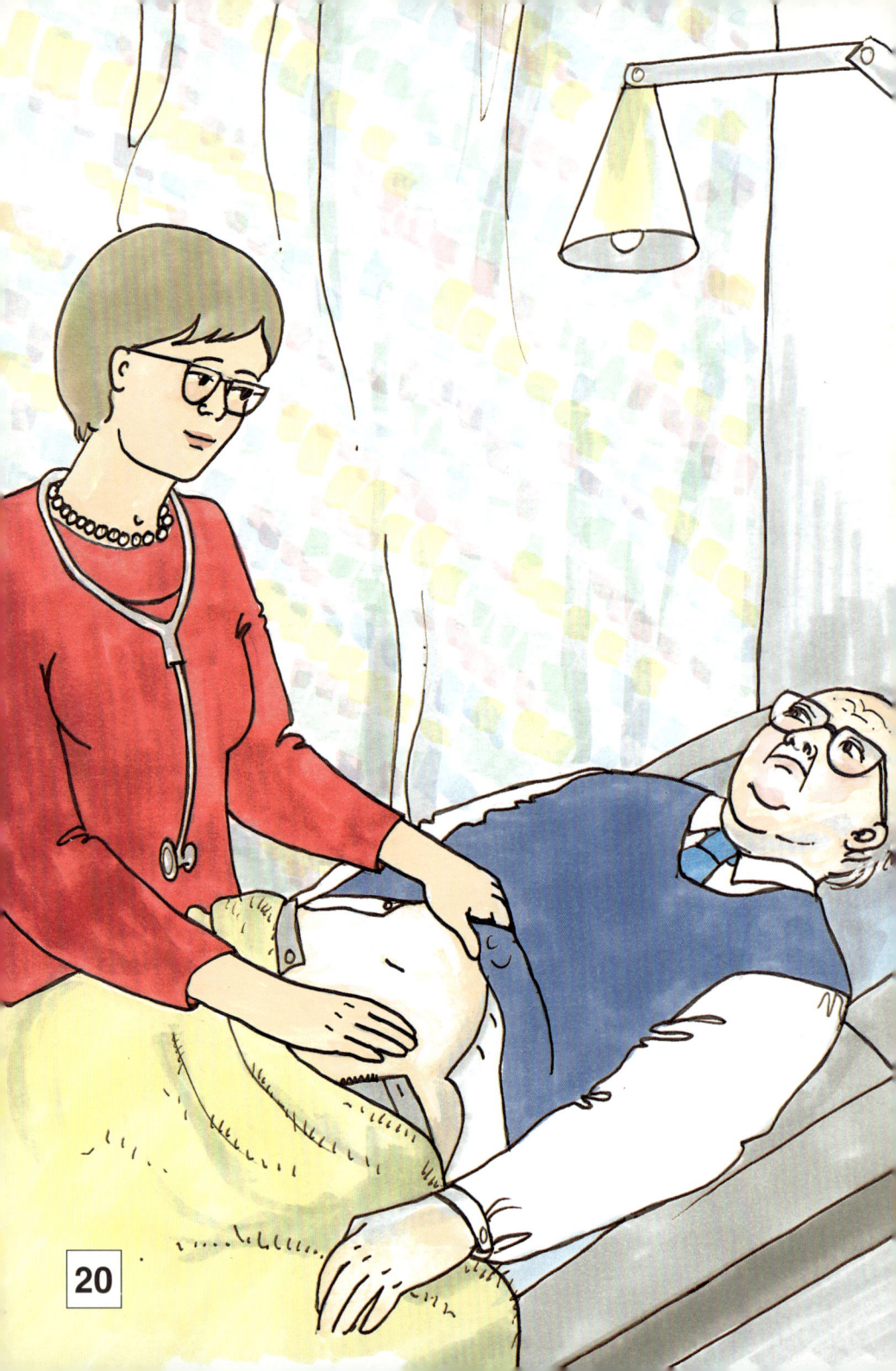

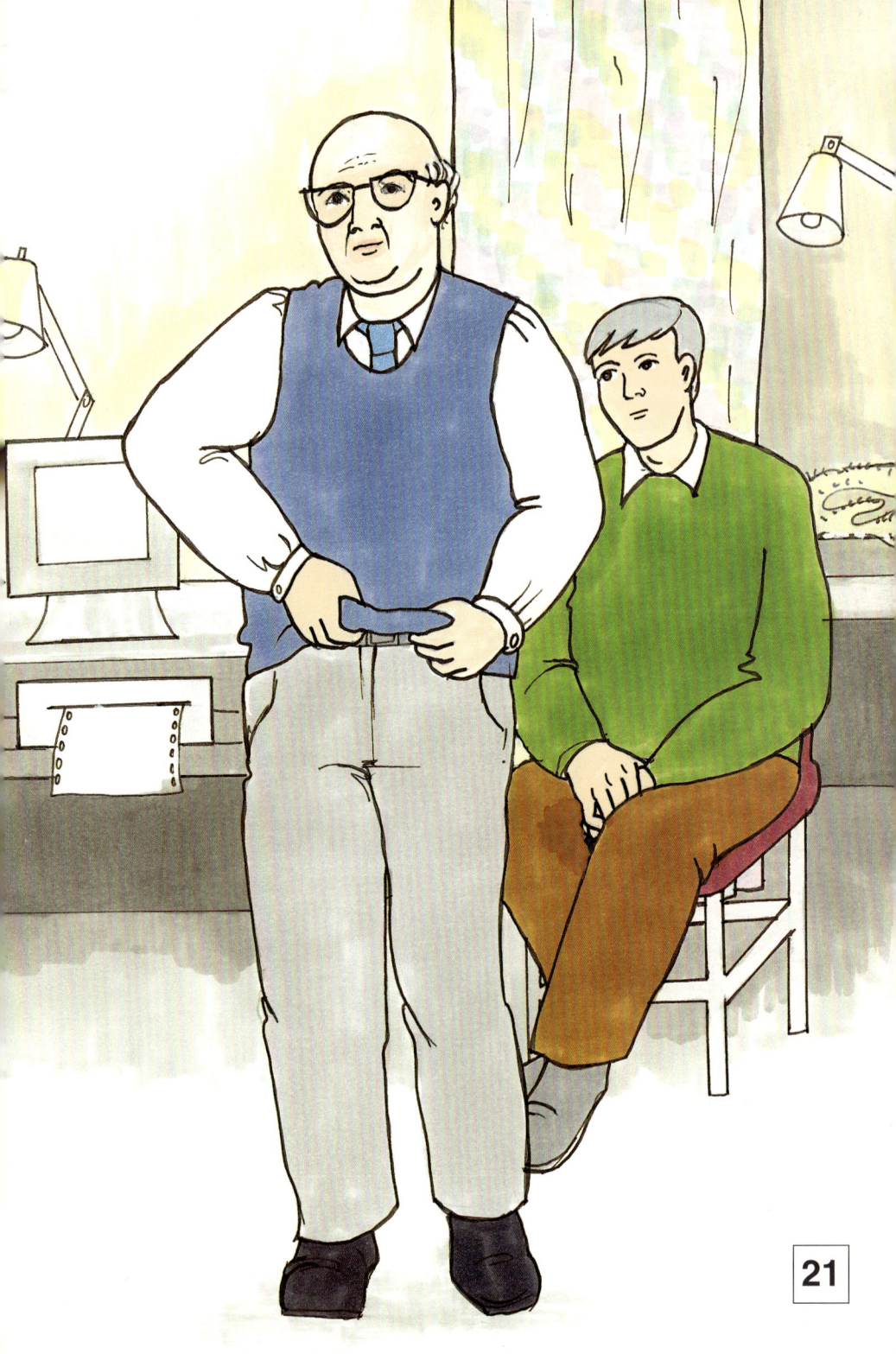

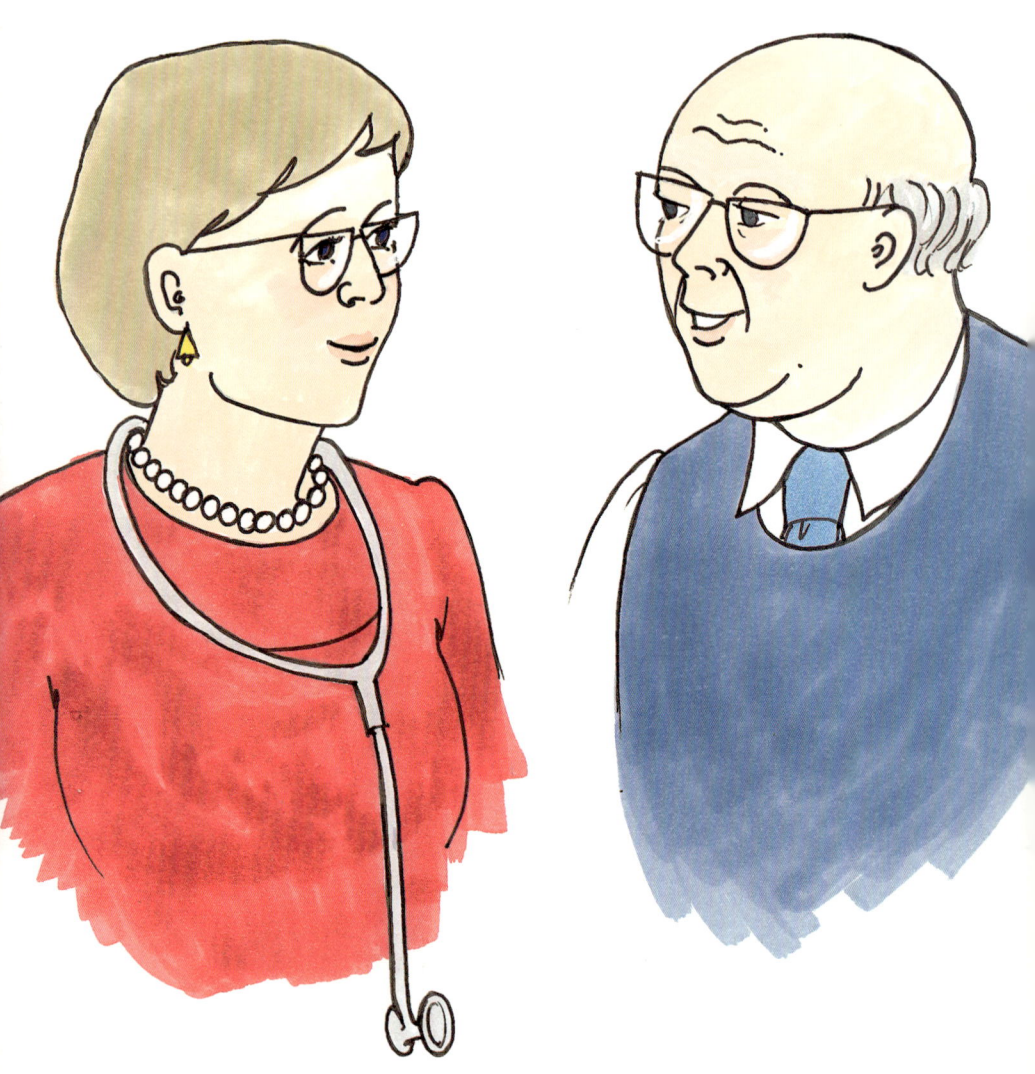

'Something hurts'

Mr Lane has an injection

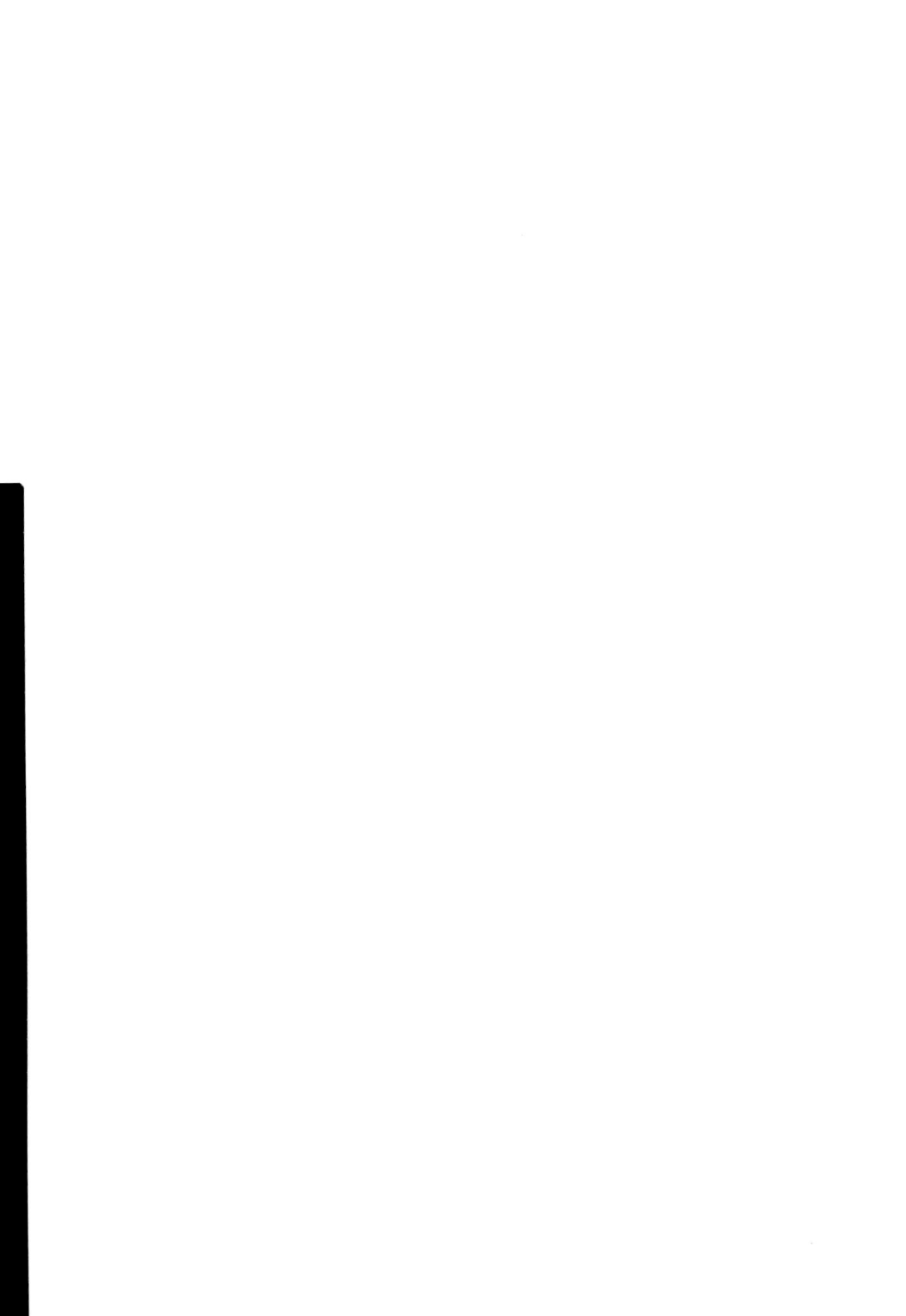

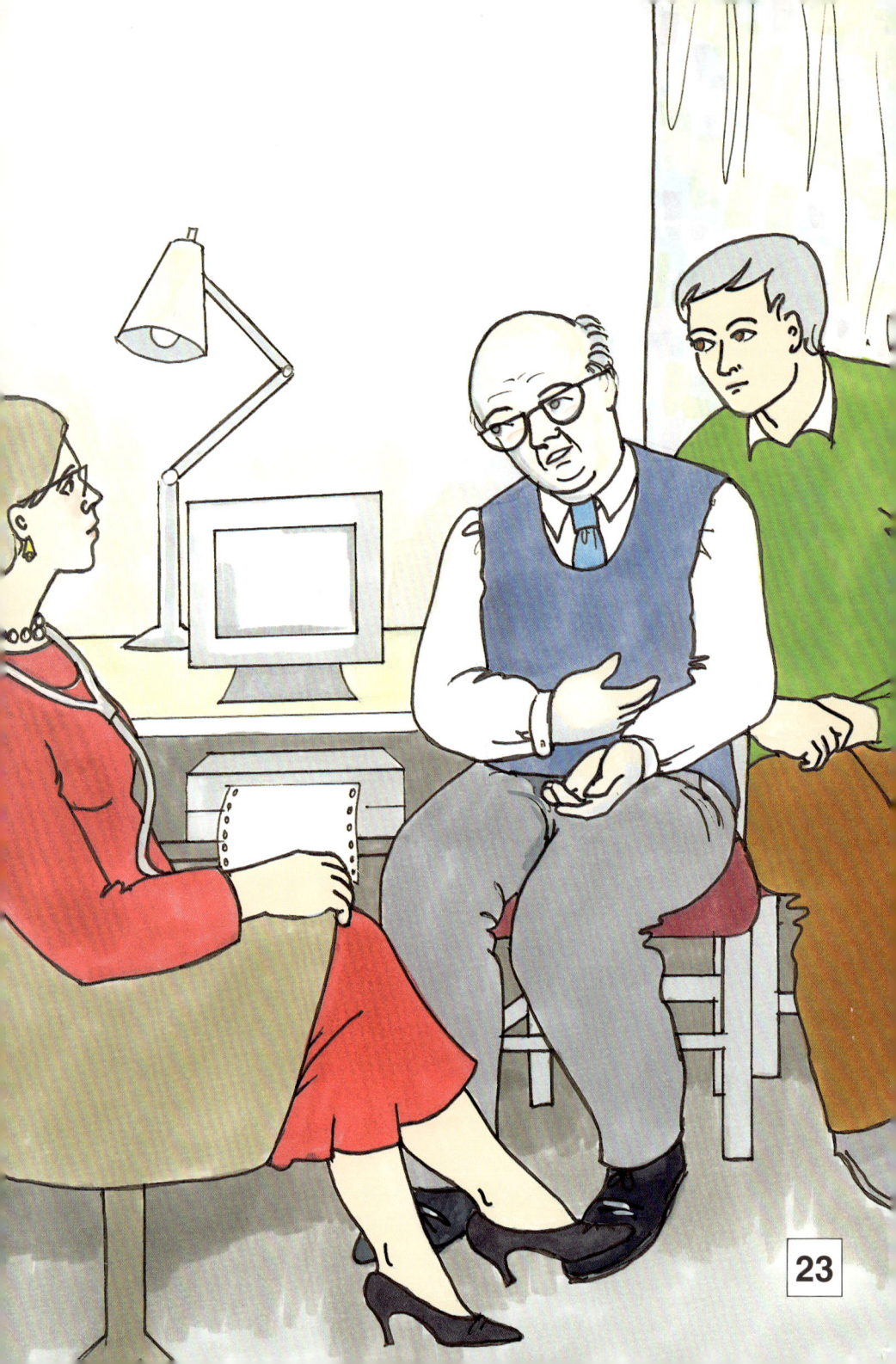

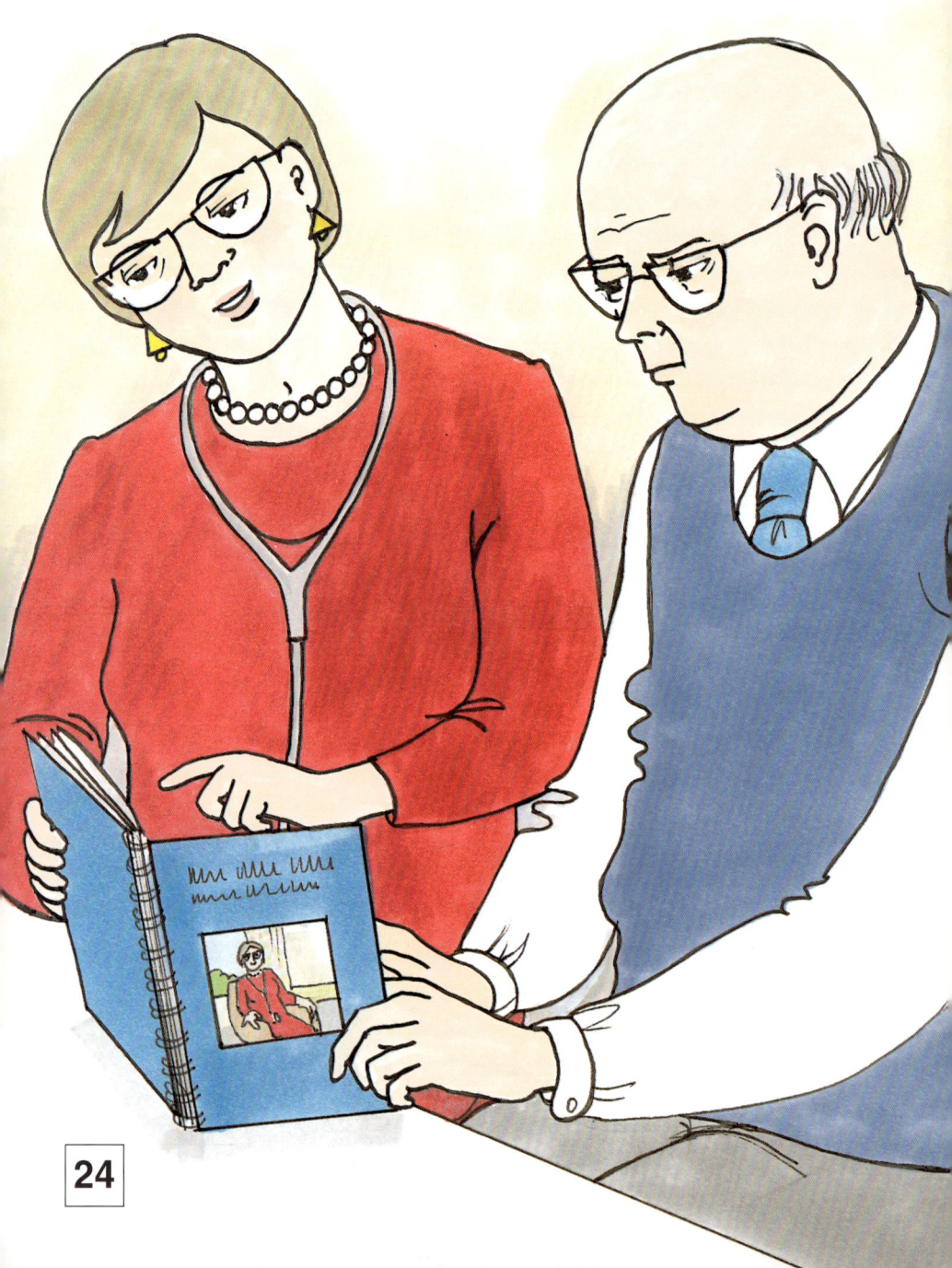

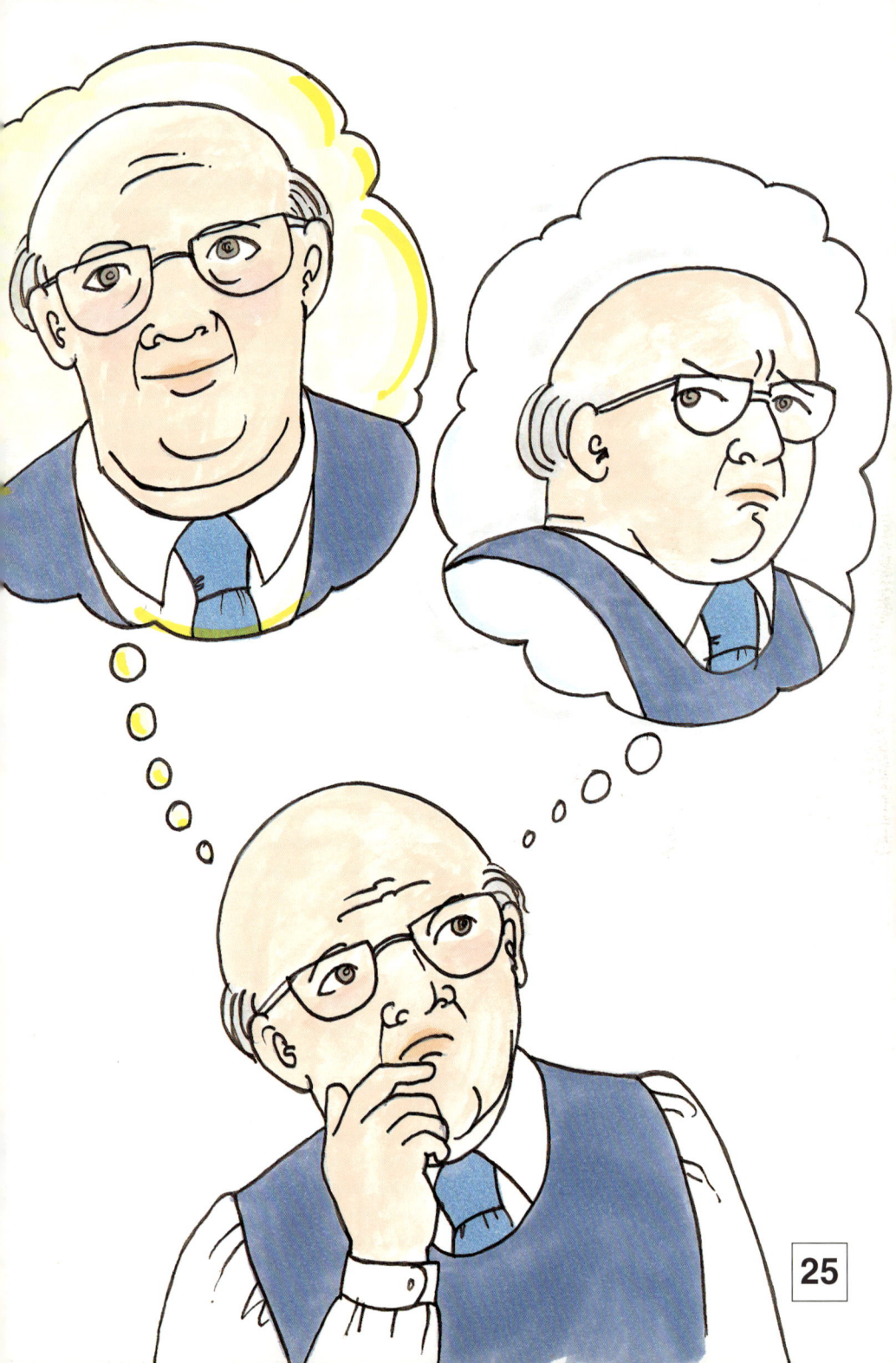

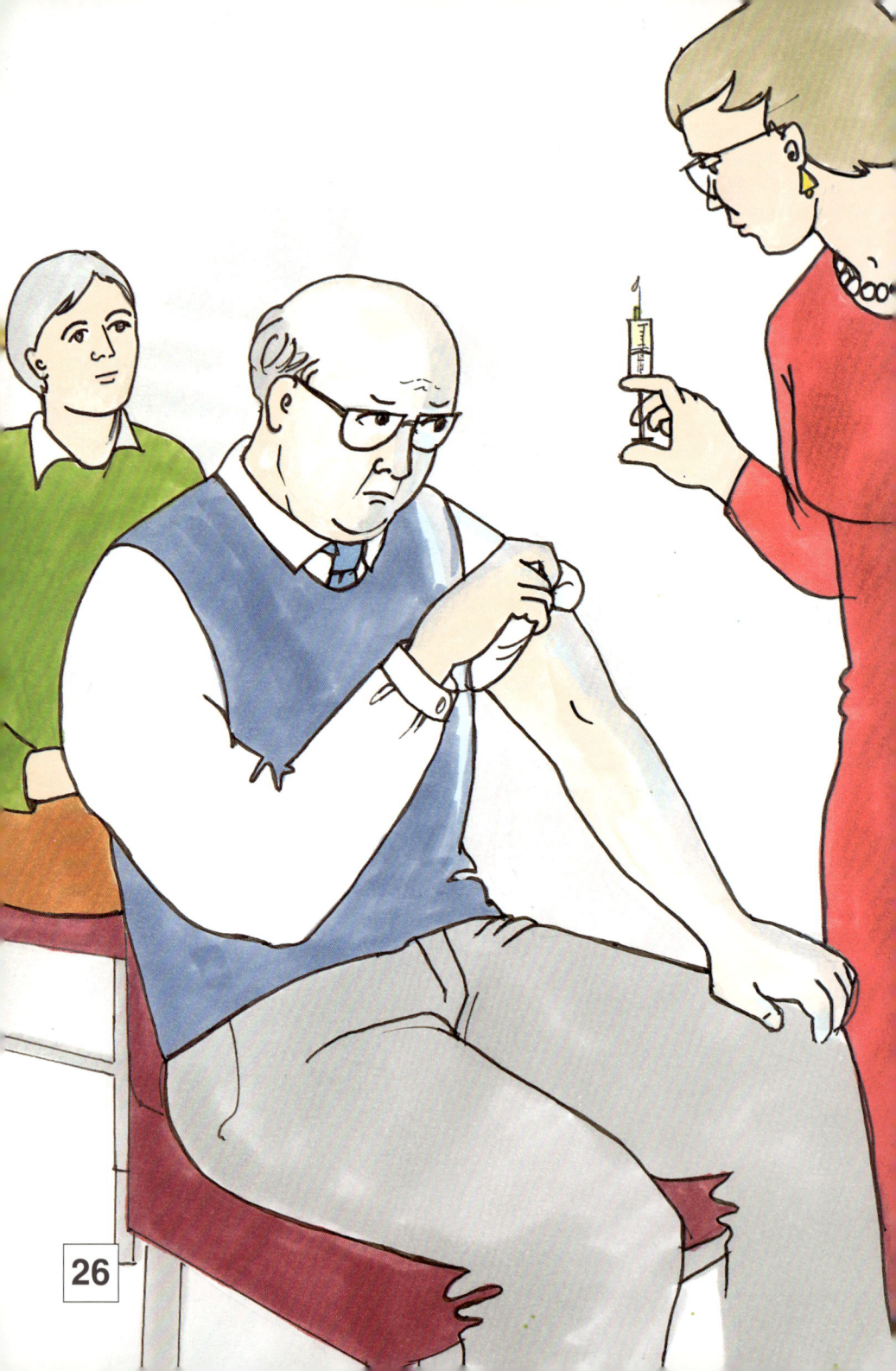

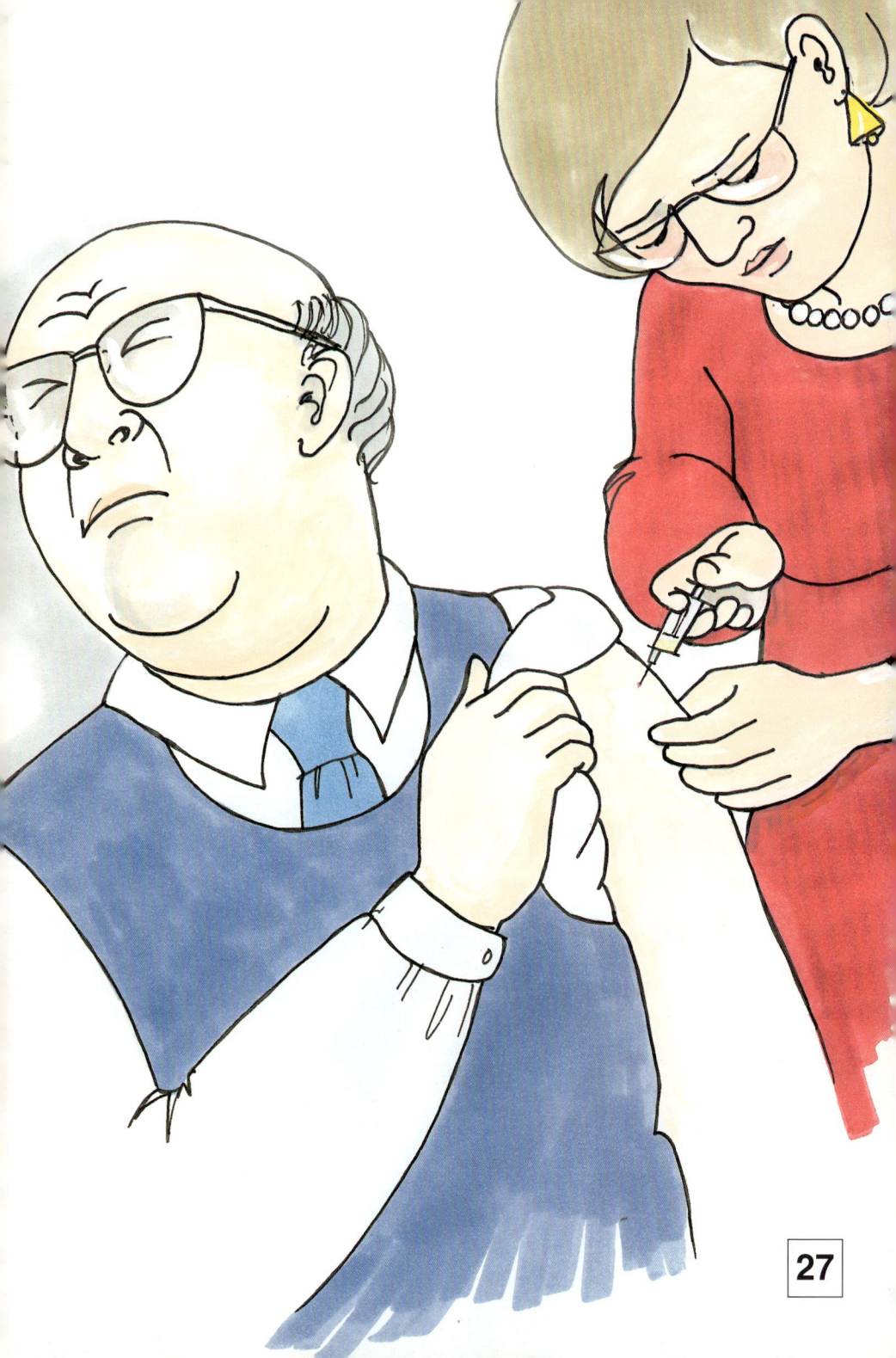

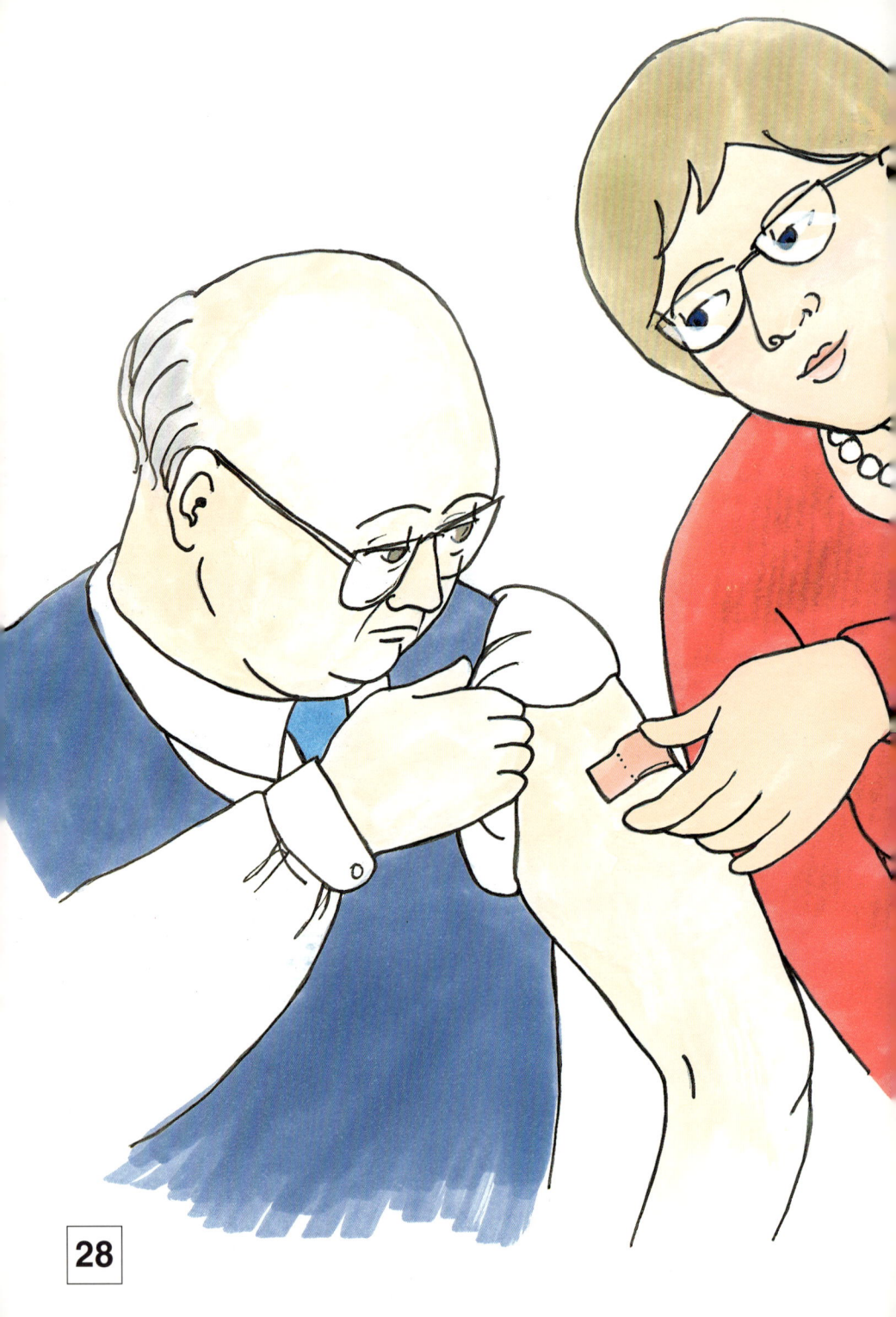

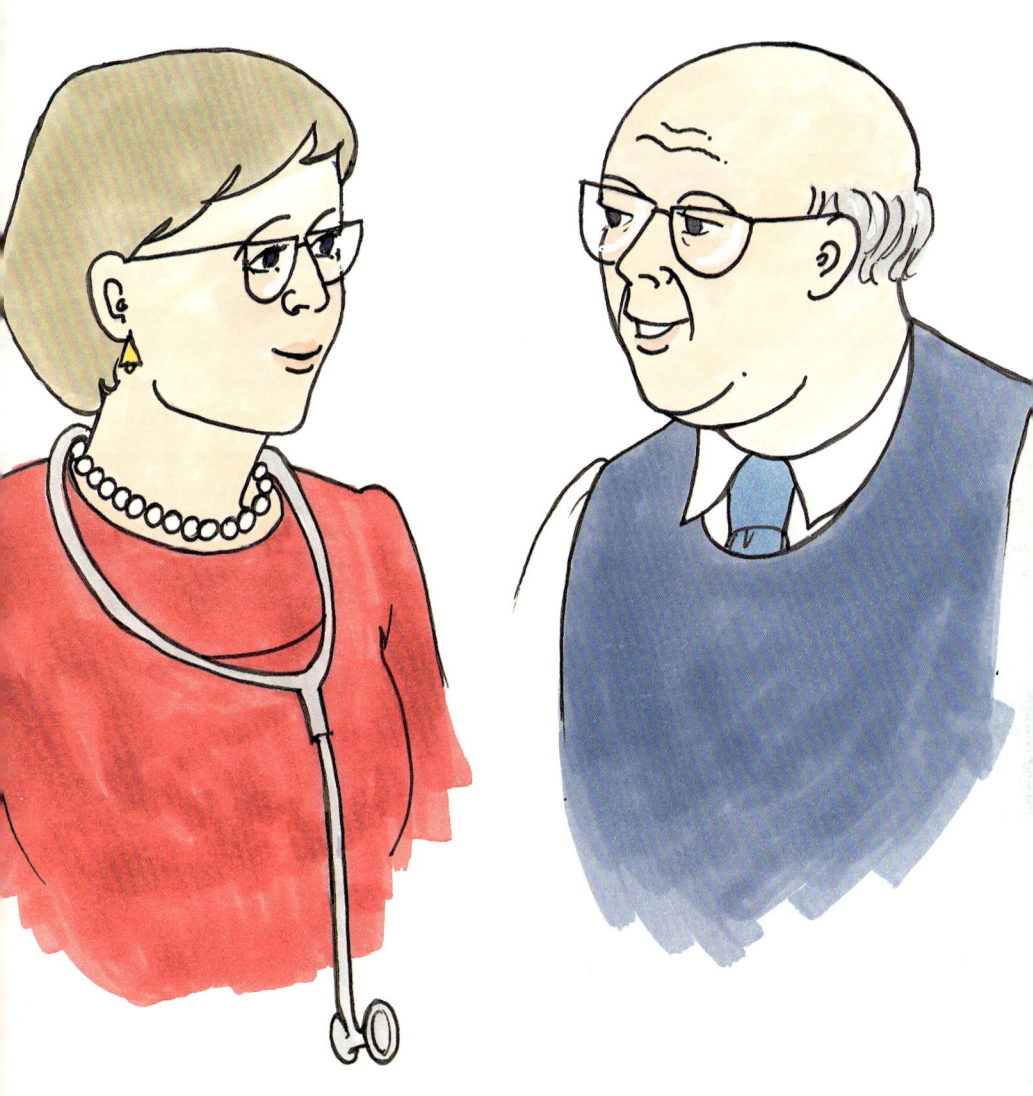

'Something makes me better'

Miss Smith has her ears syringed

4: Ears Syringed

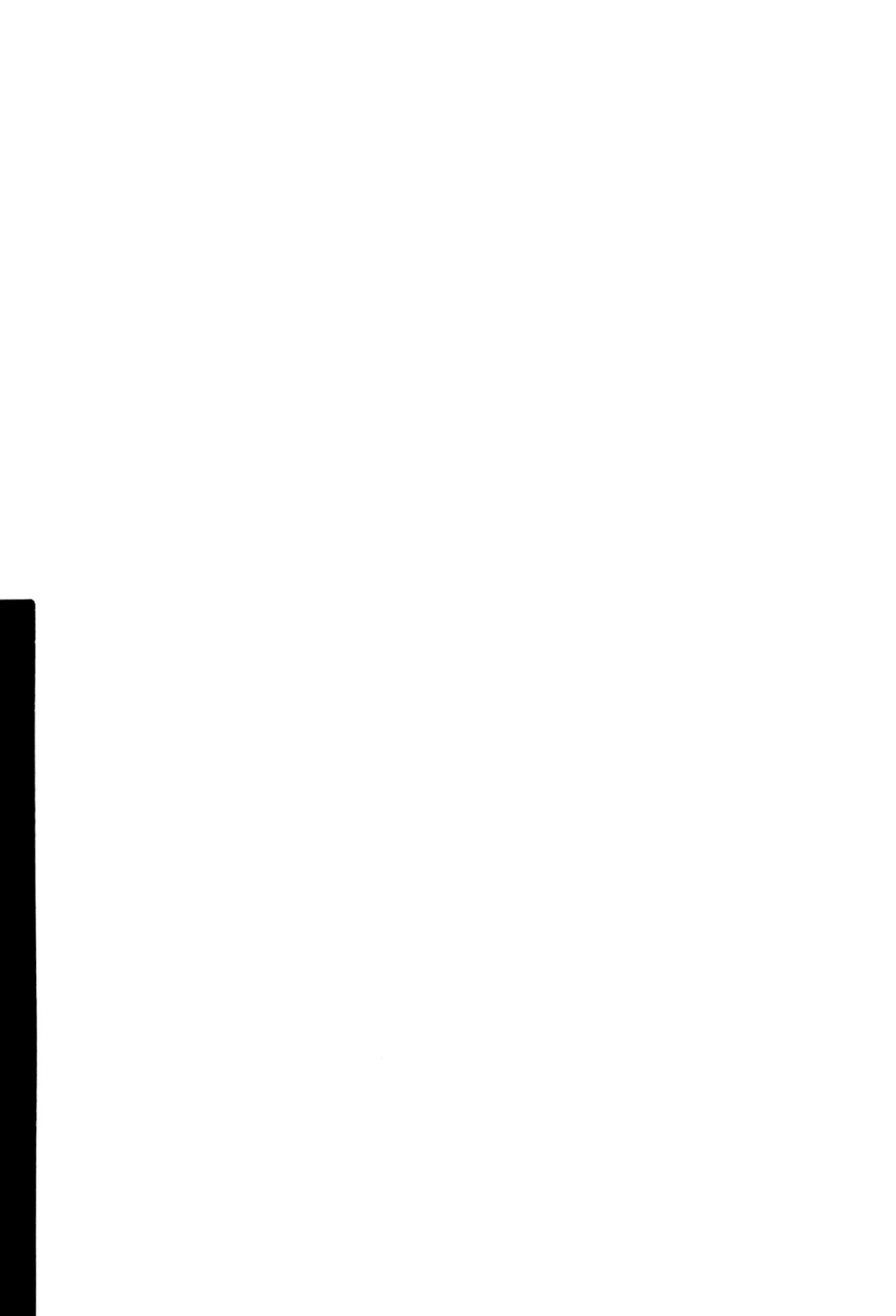

10:34

Dr

30

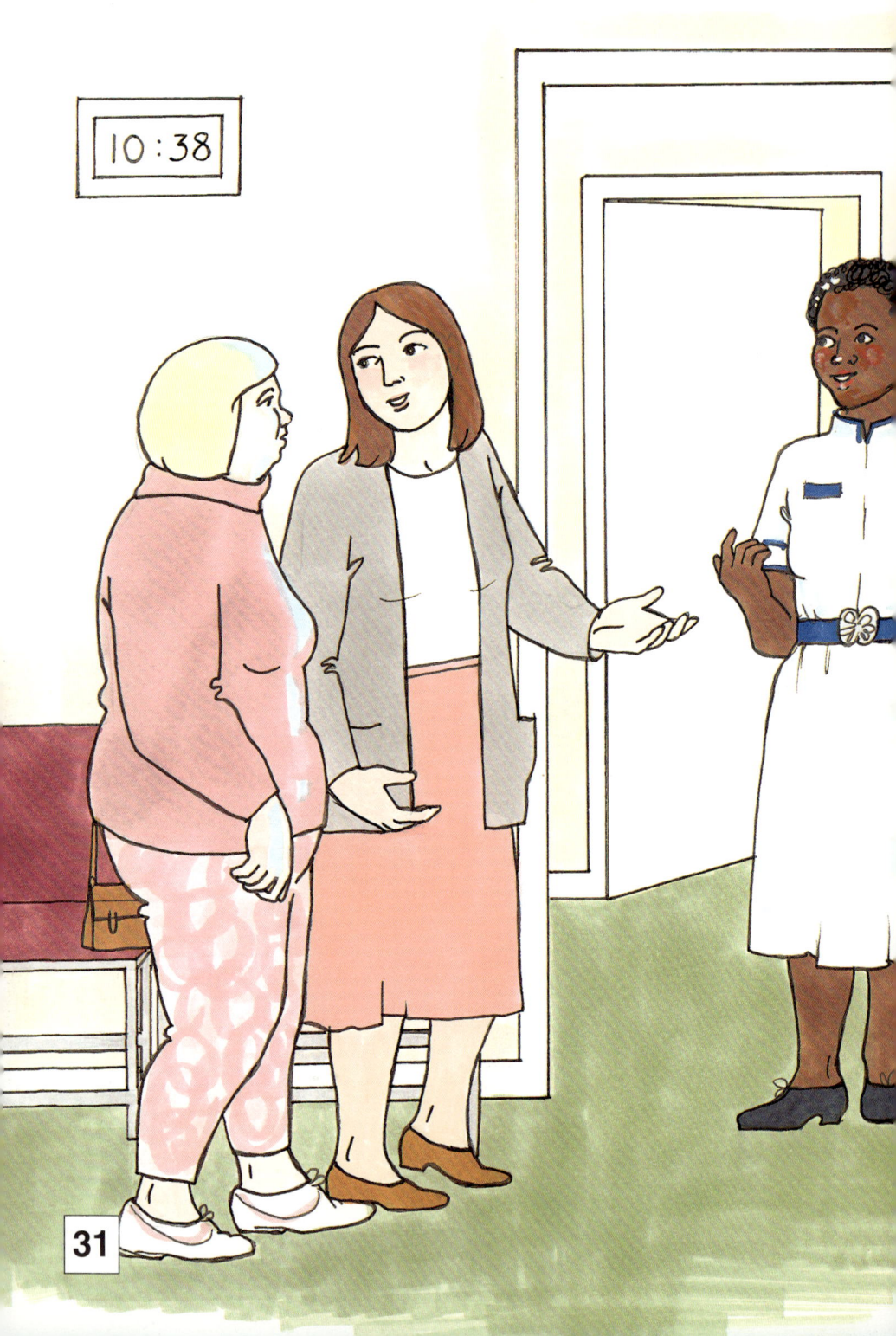

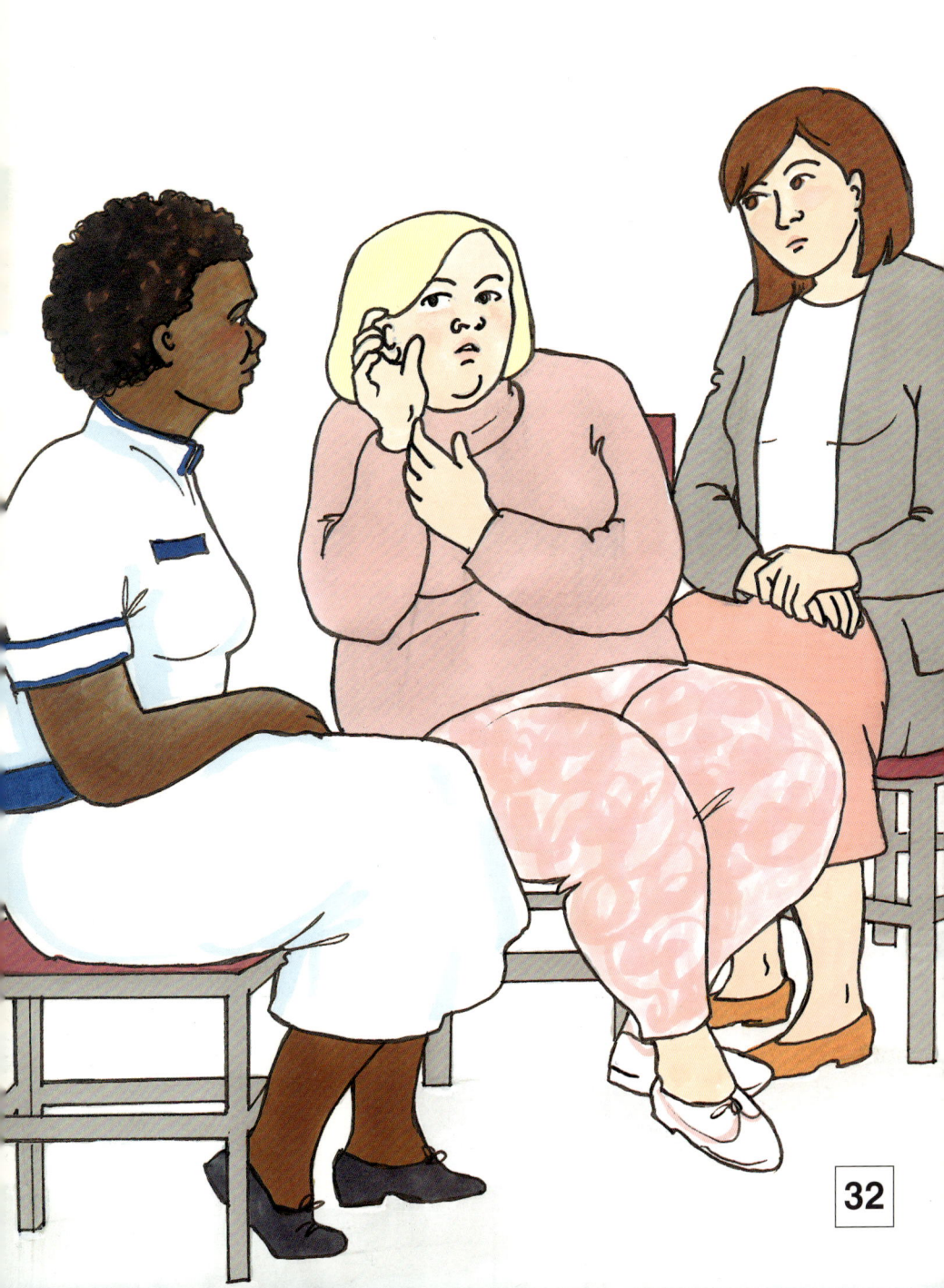

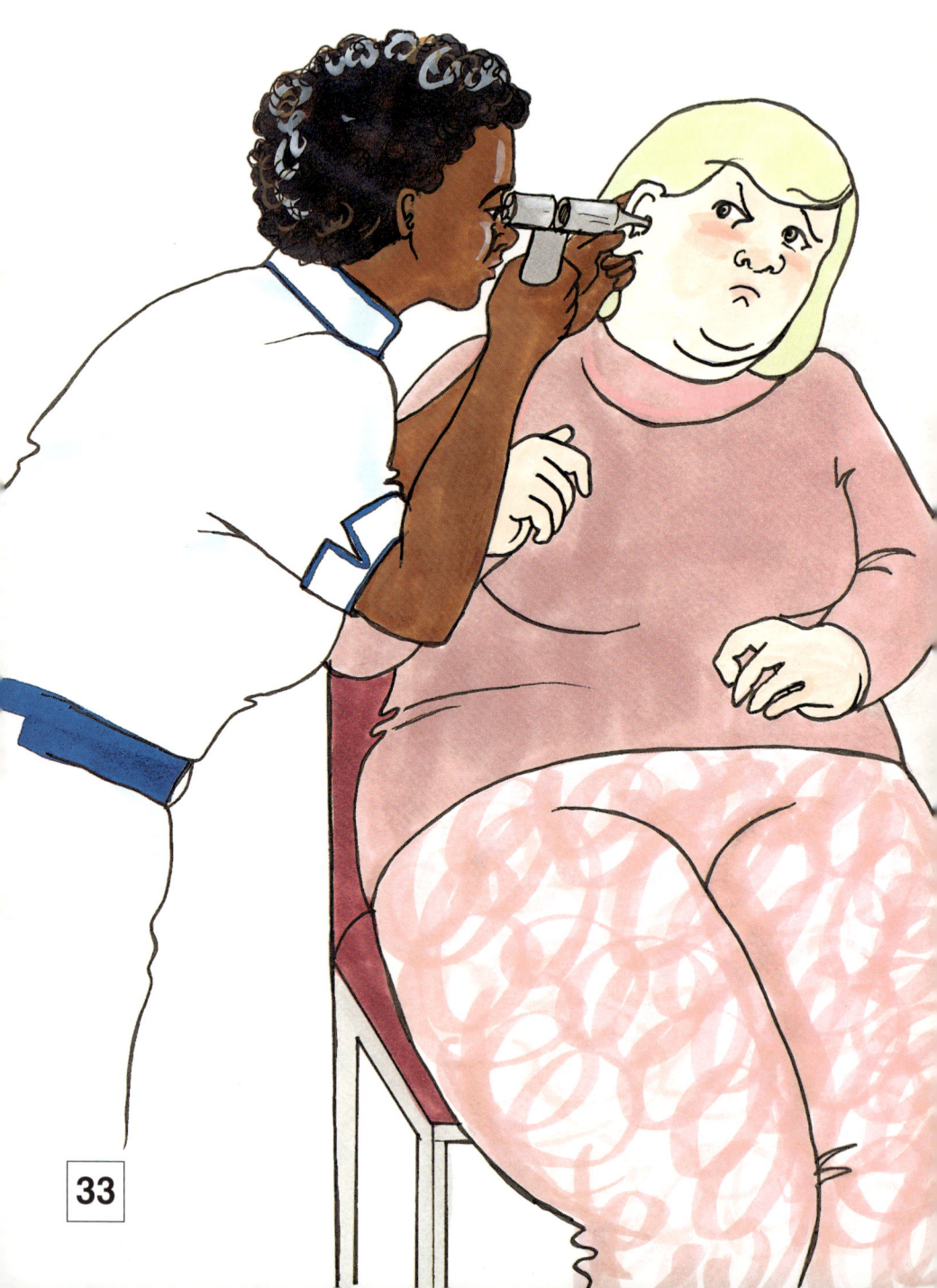

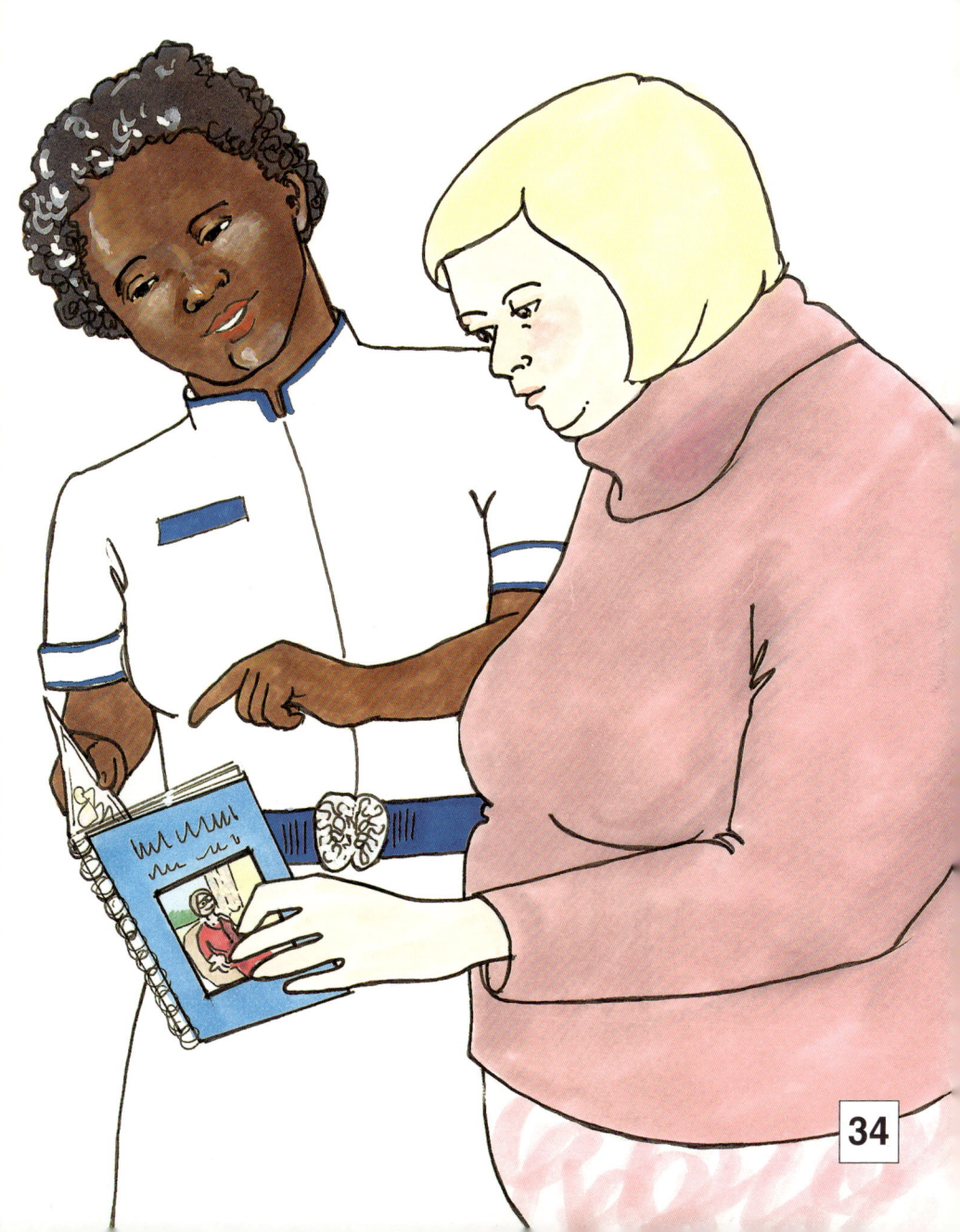

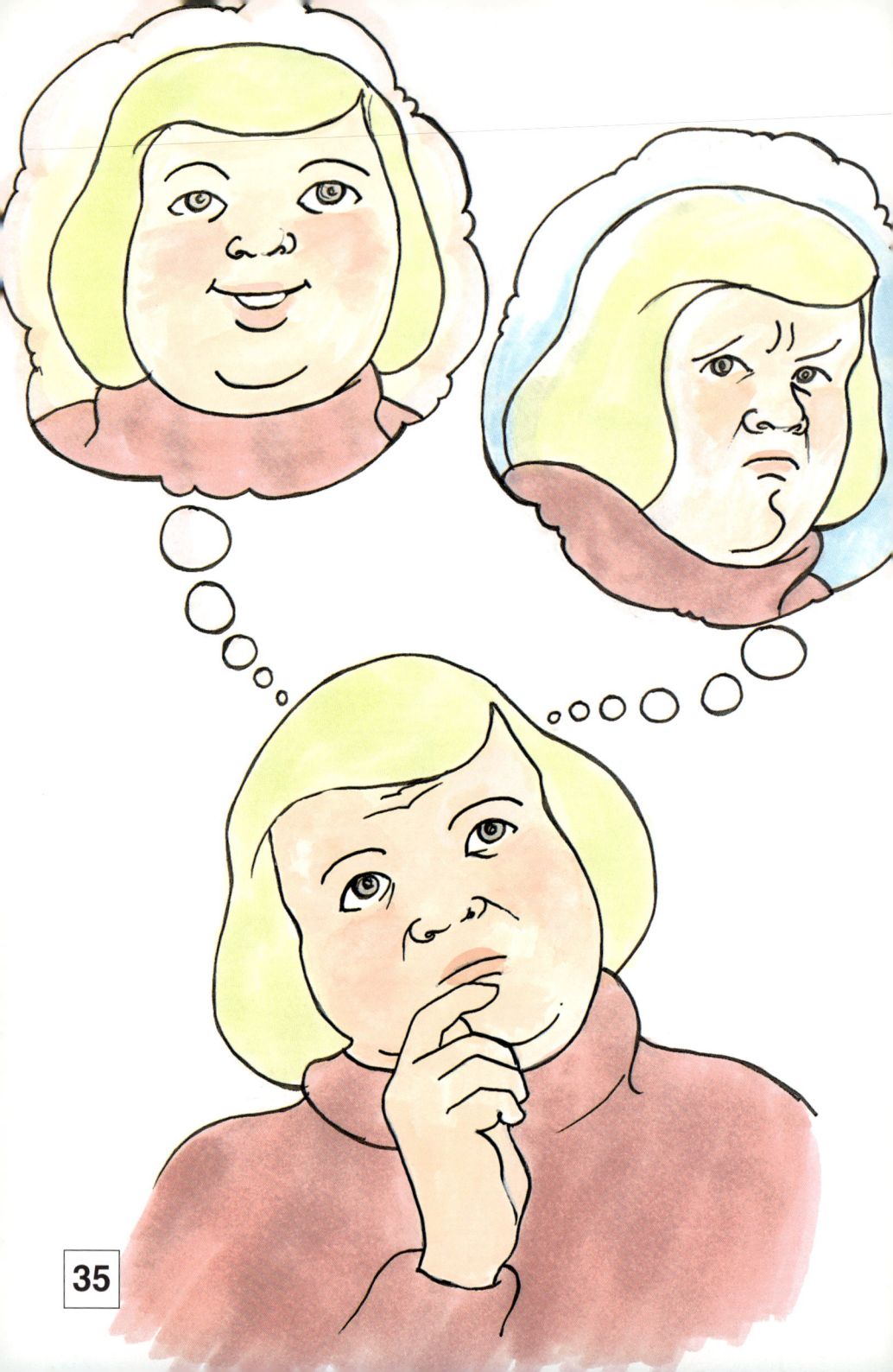

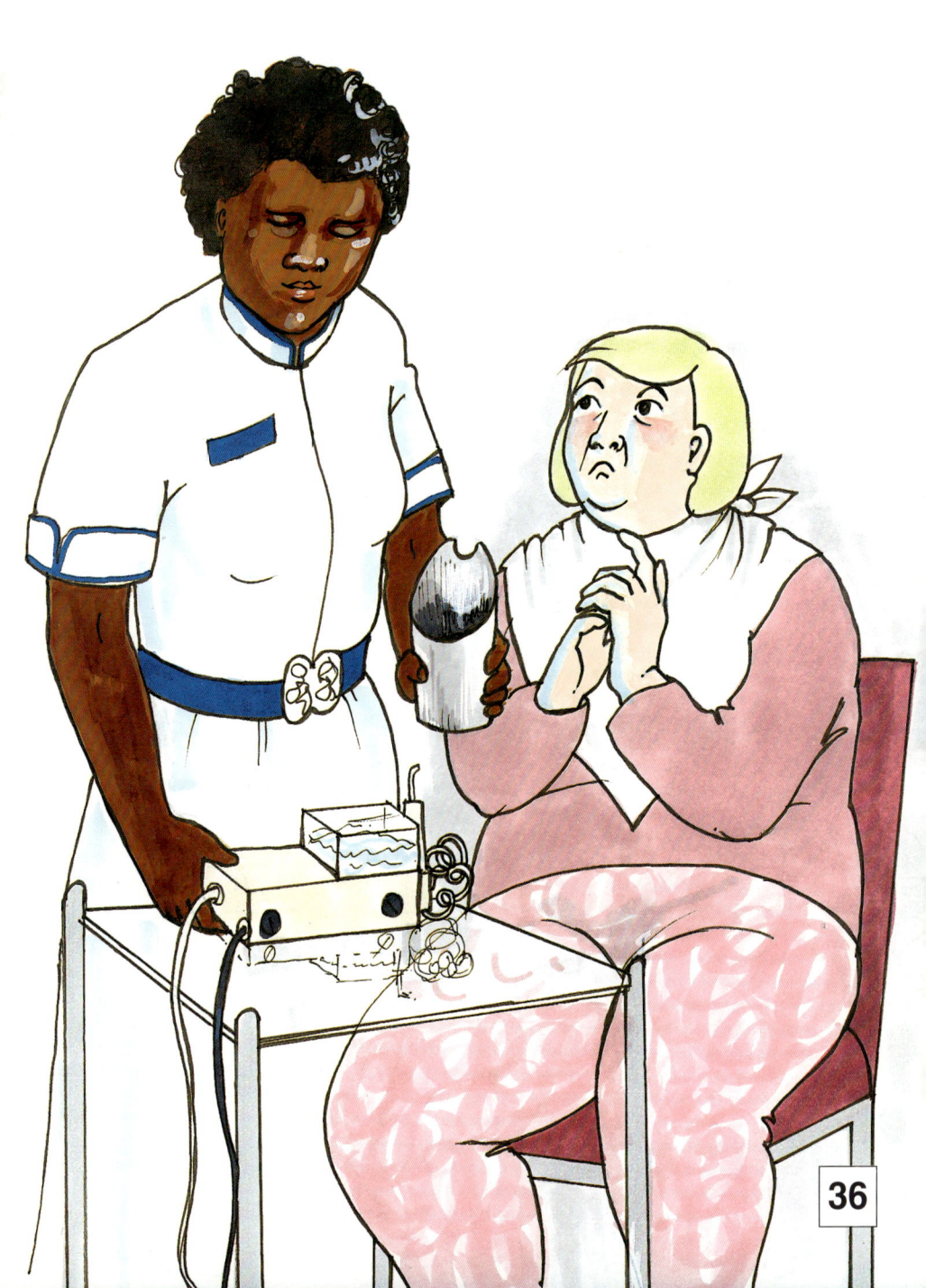

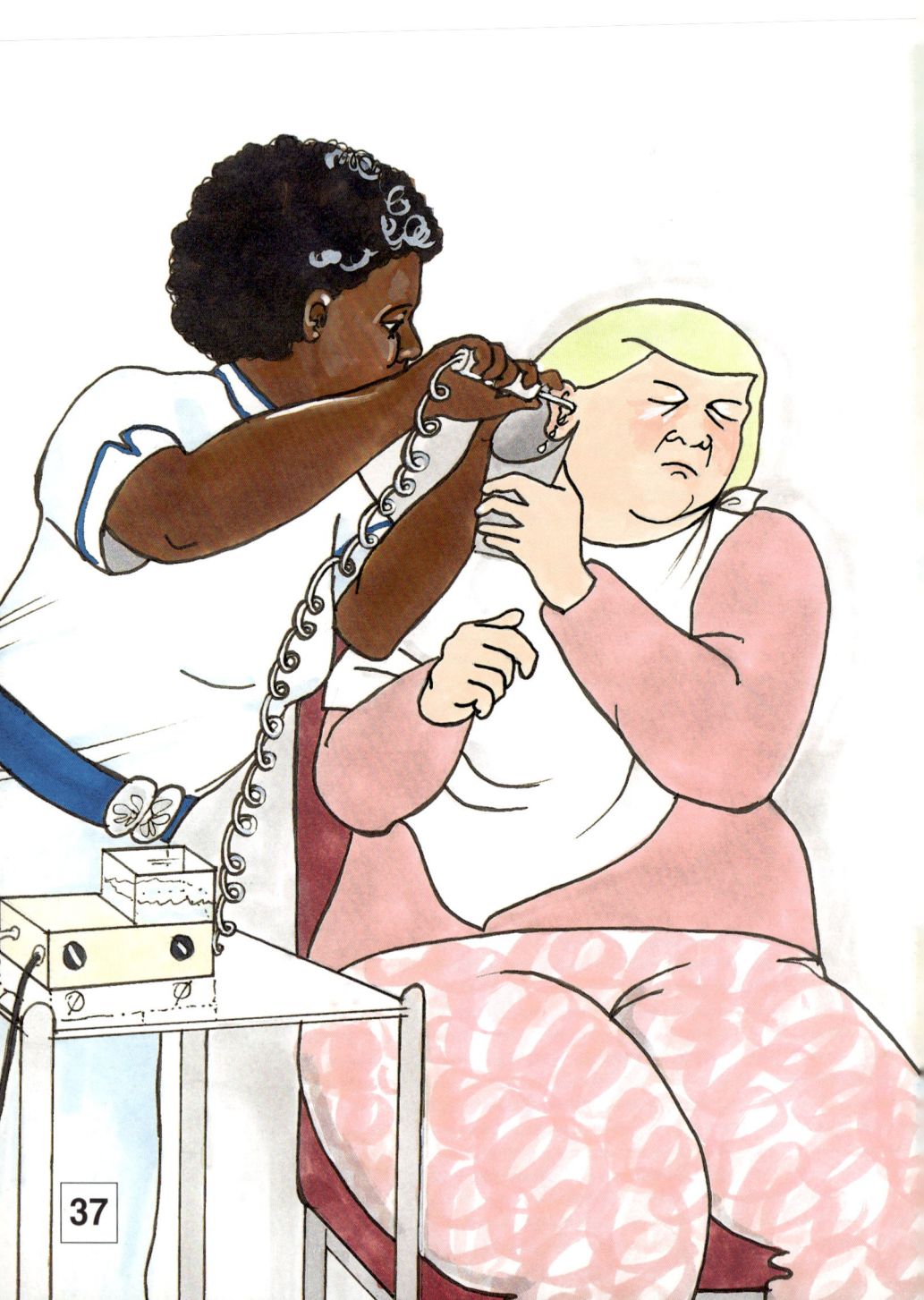

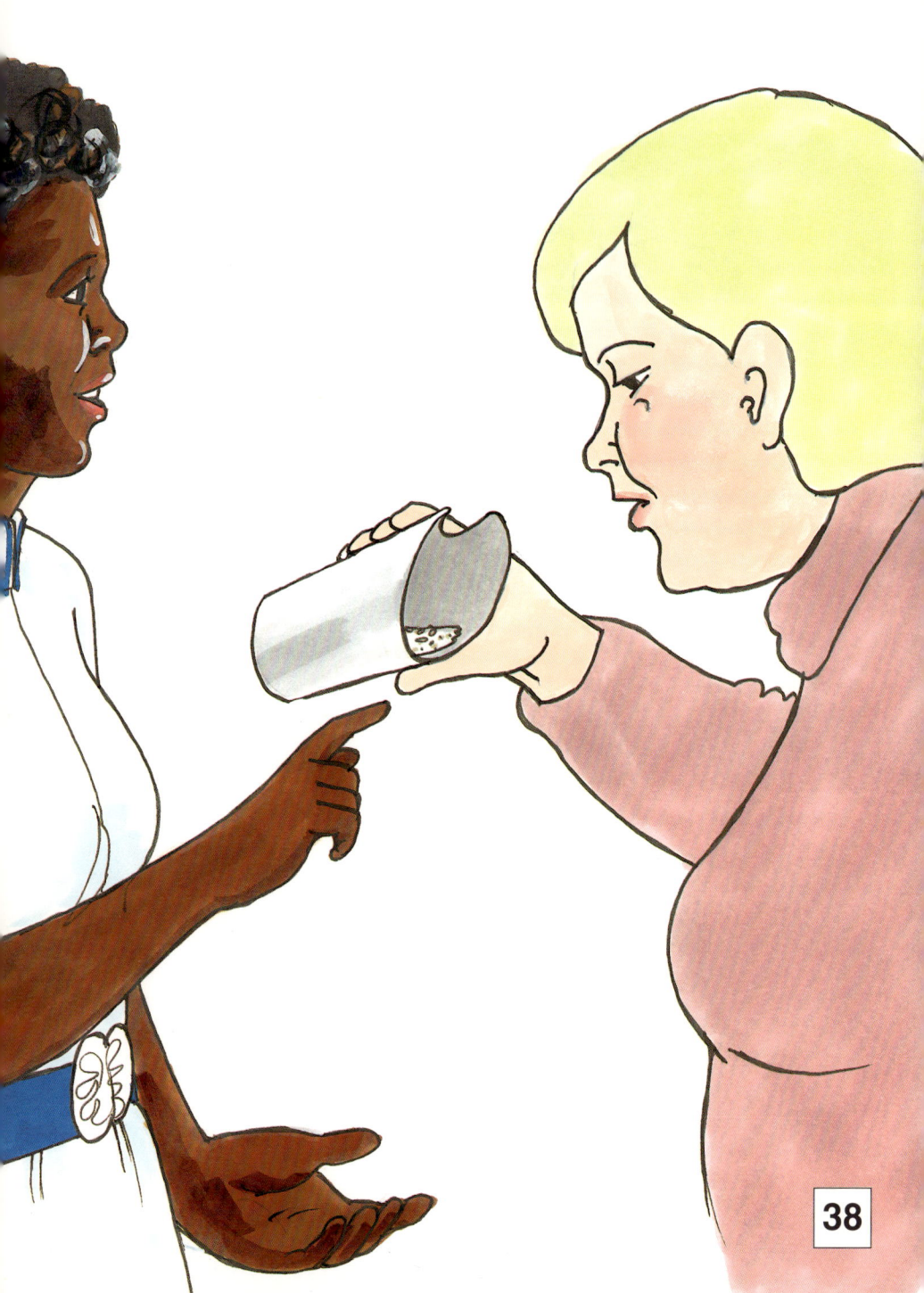

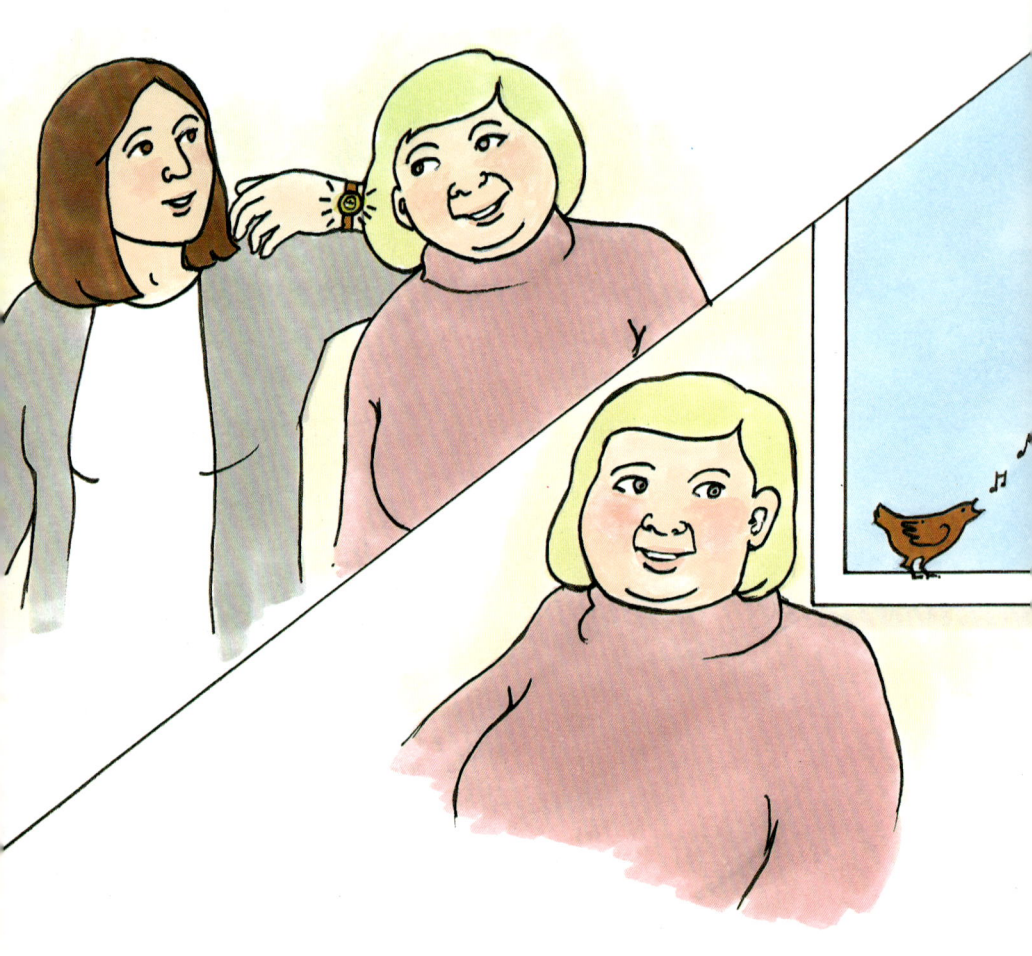

'Something pricks'

Miss Smith has a blood test

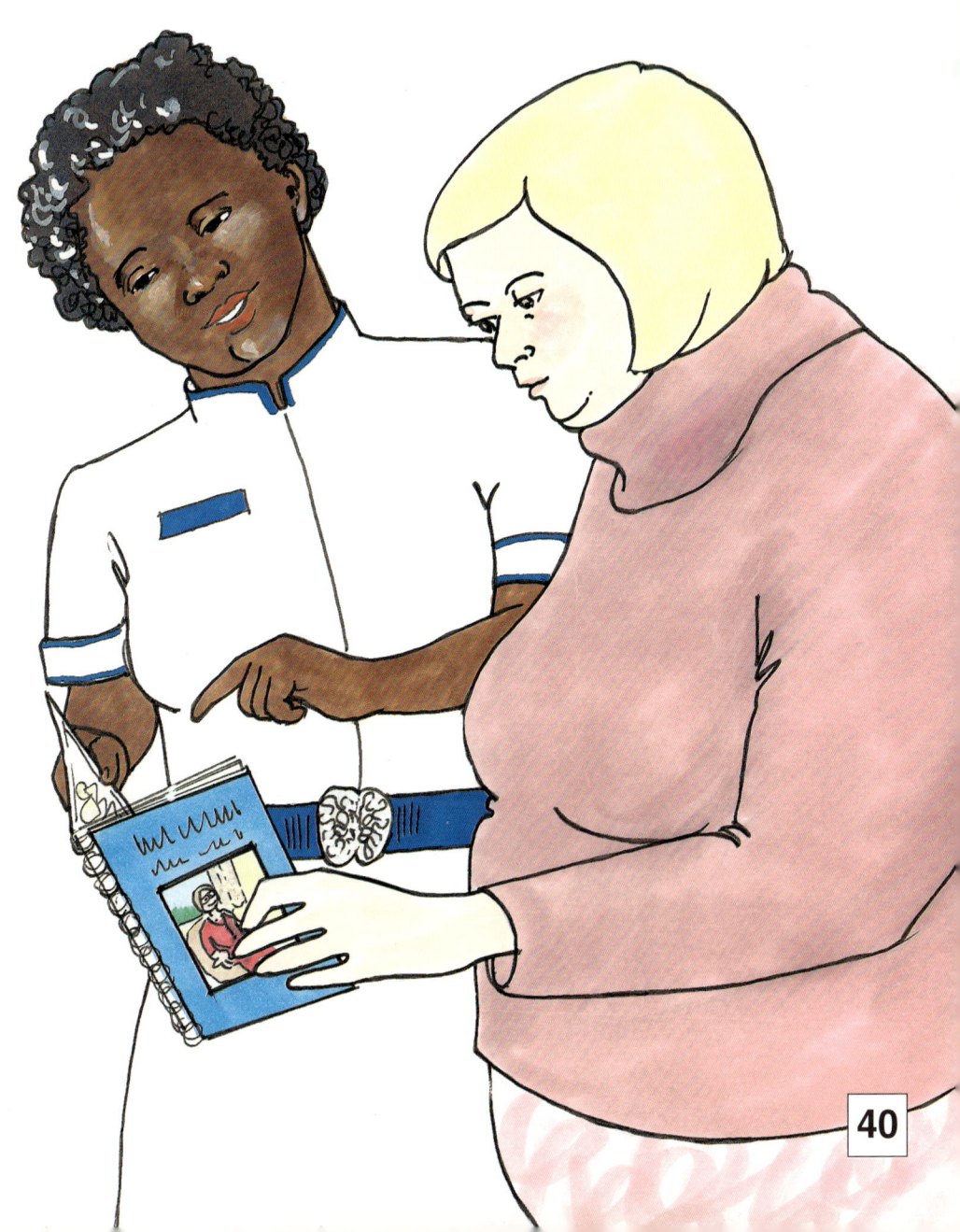

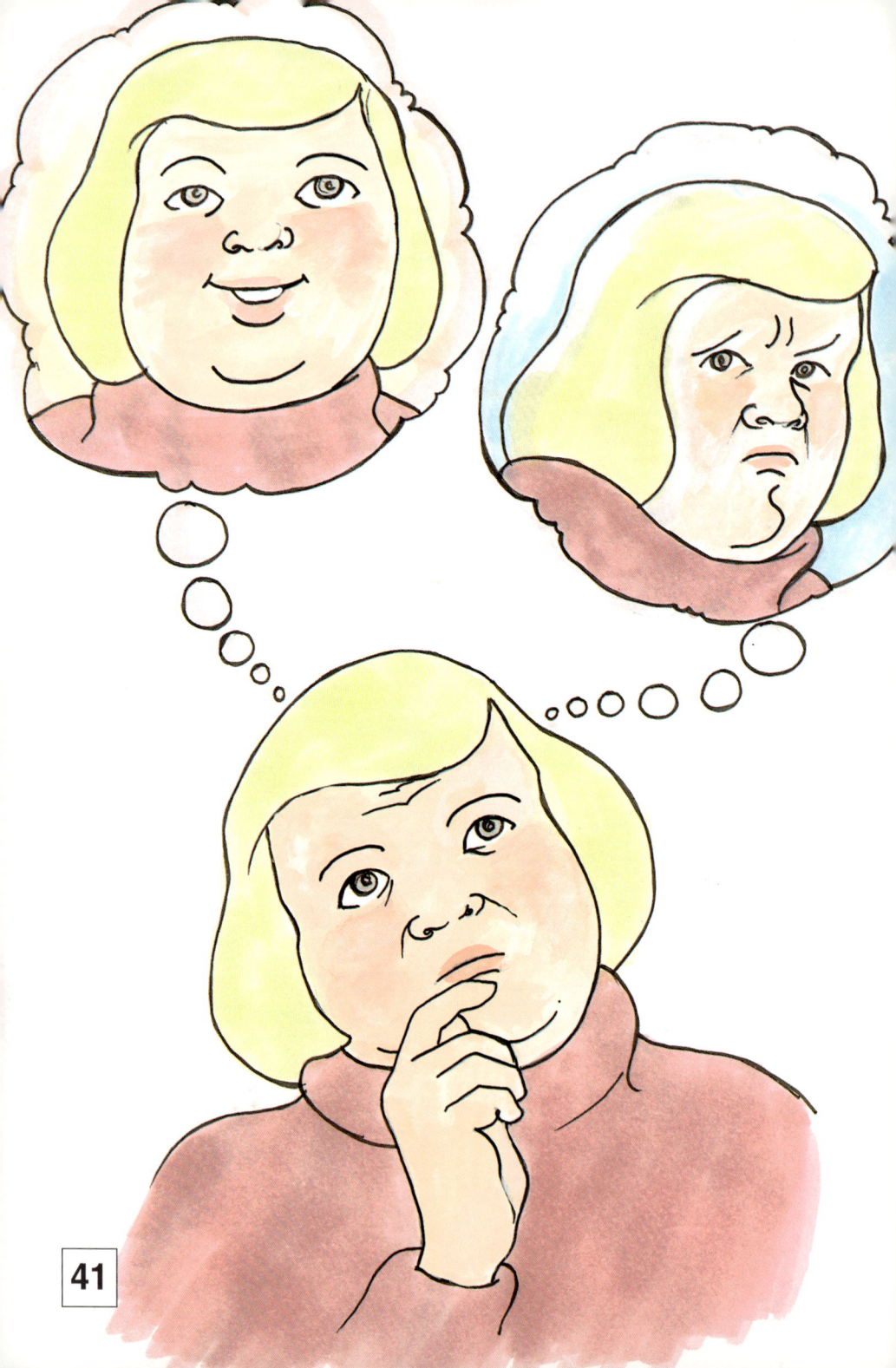

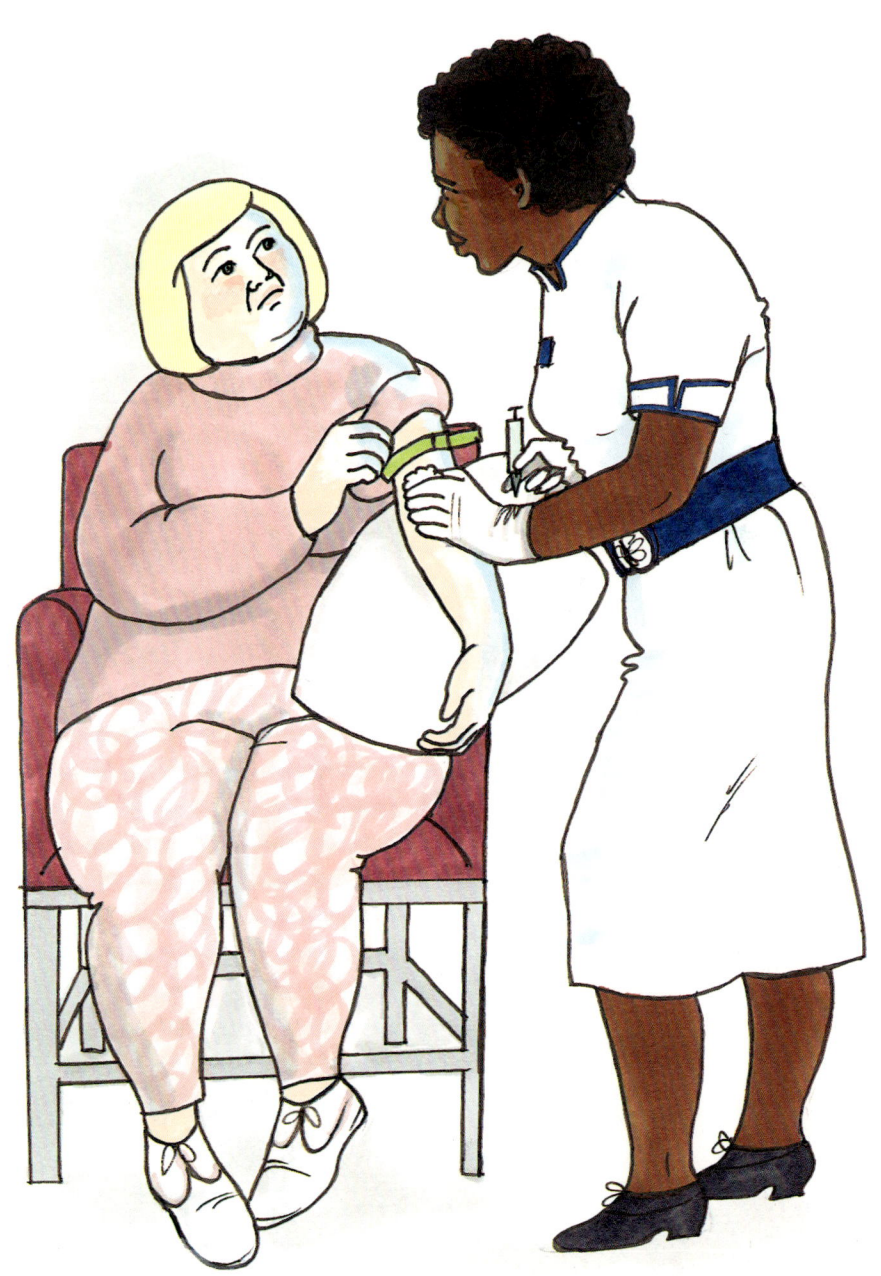

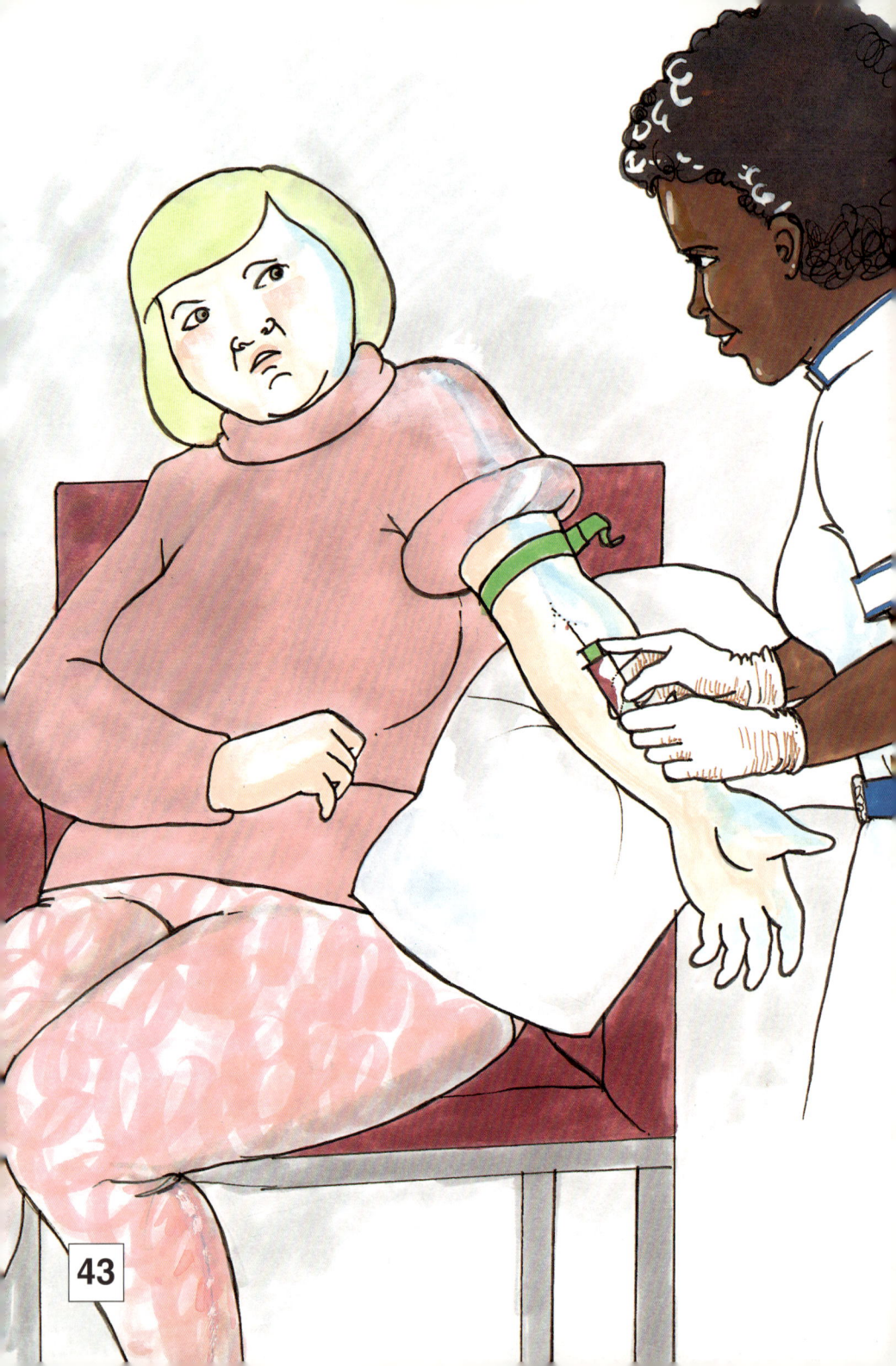

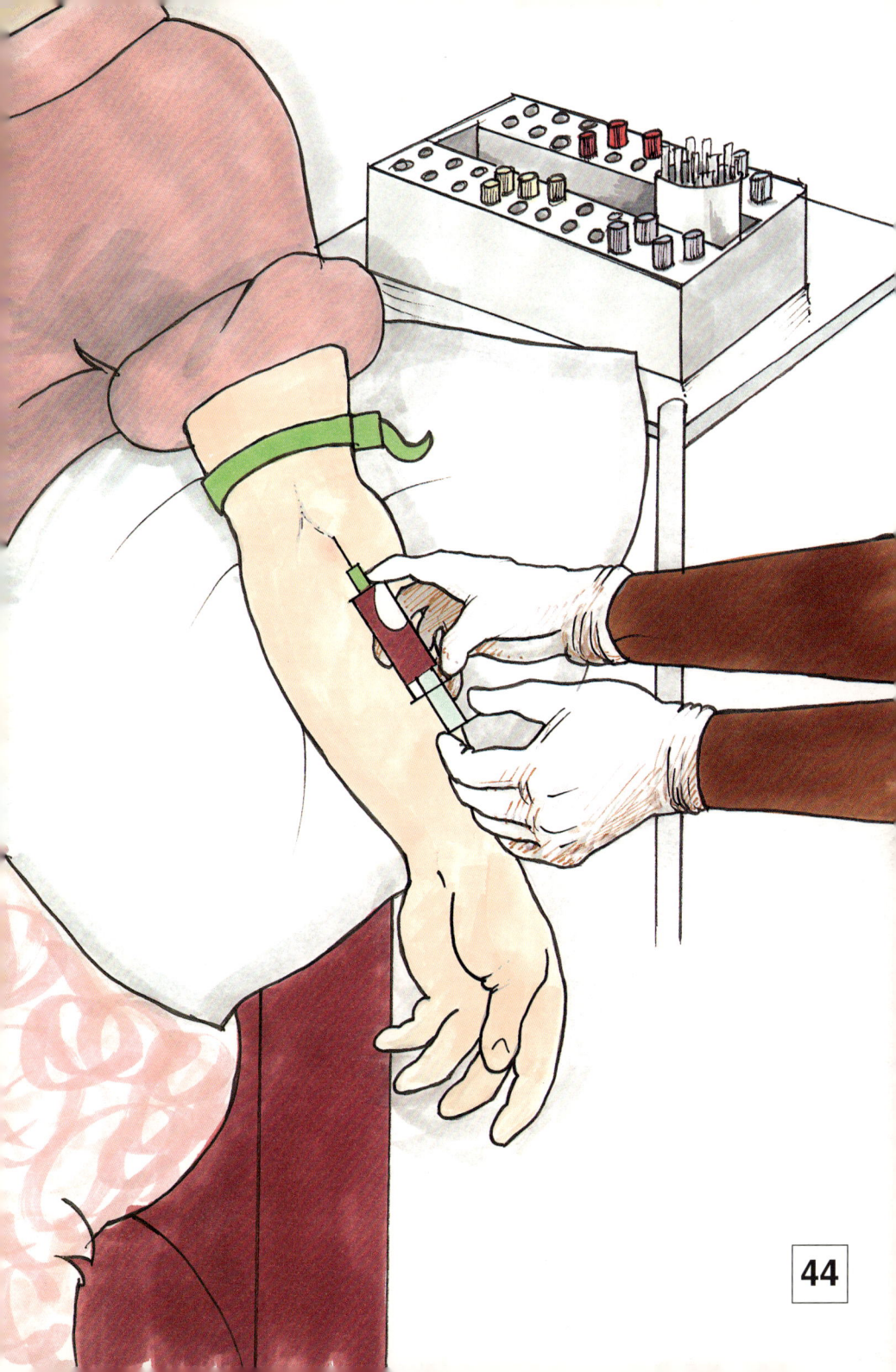

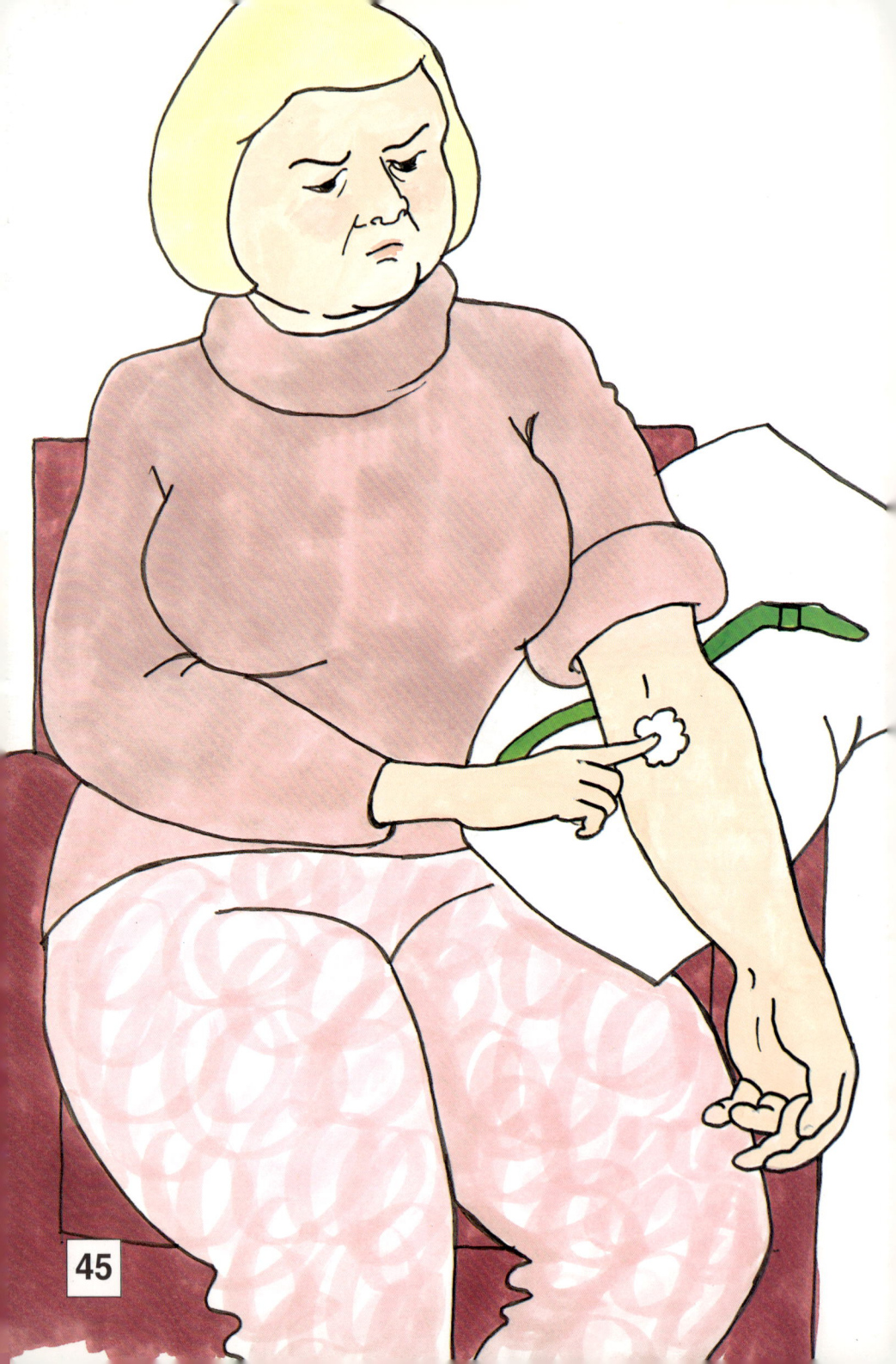

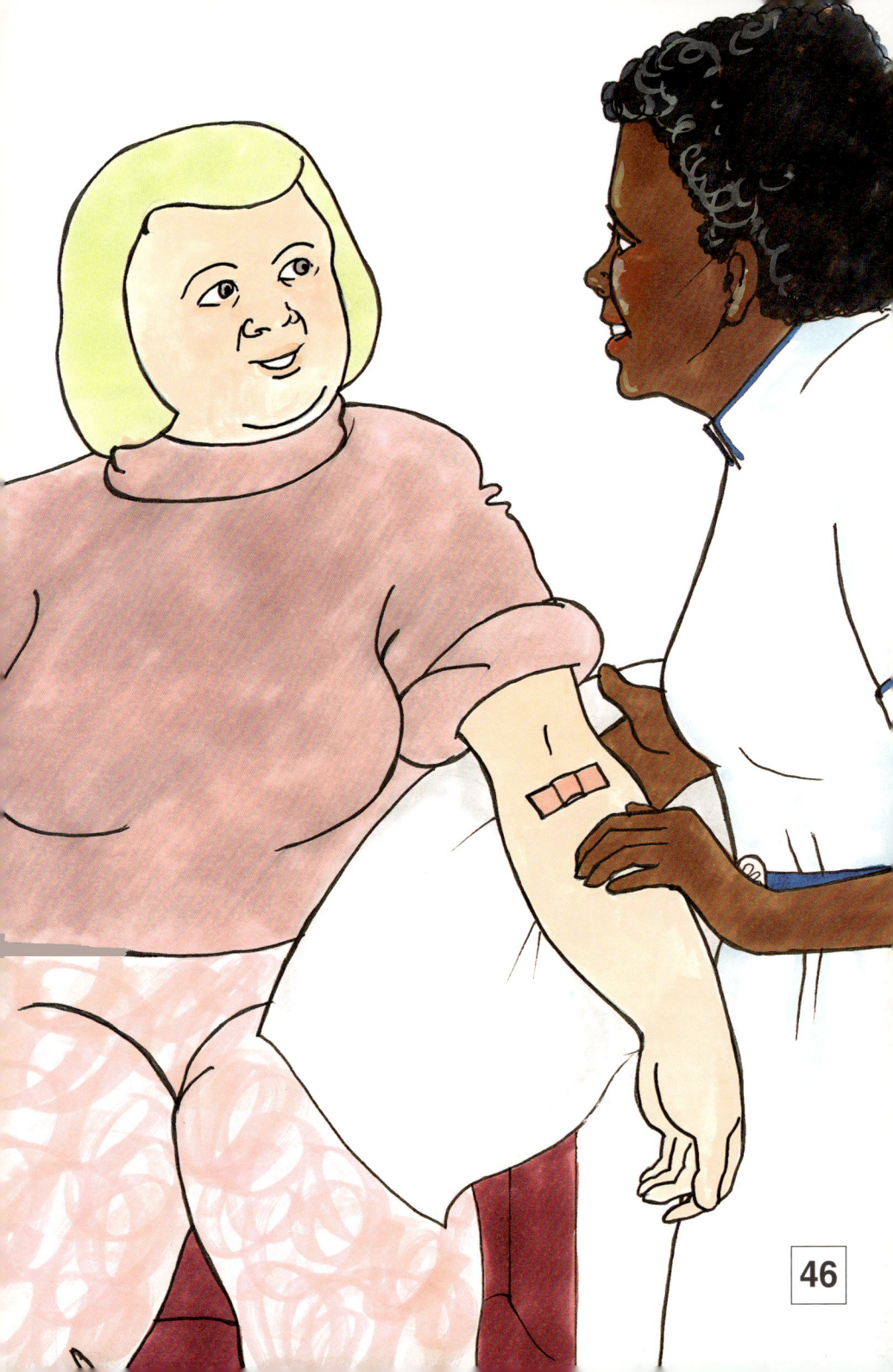

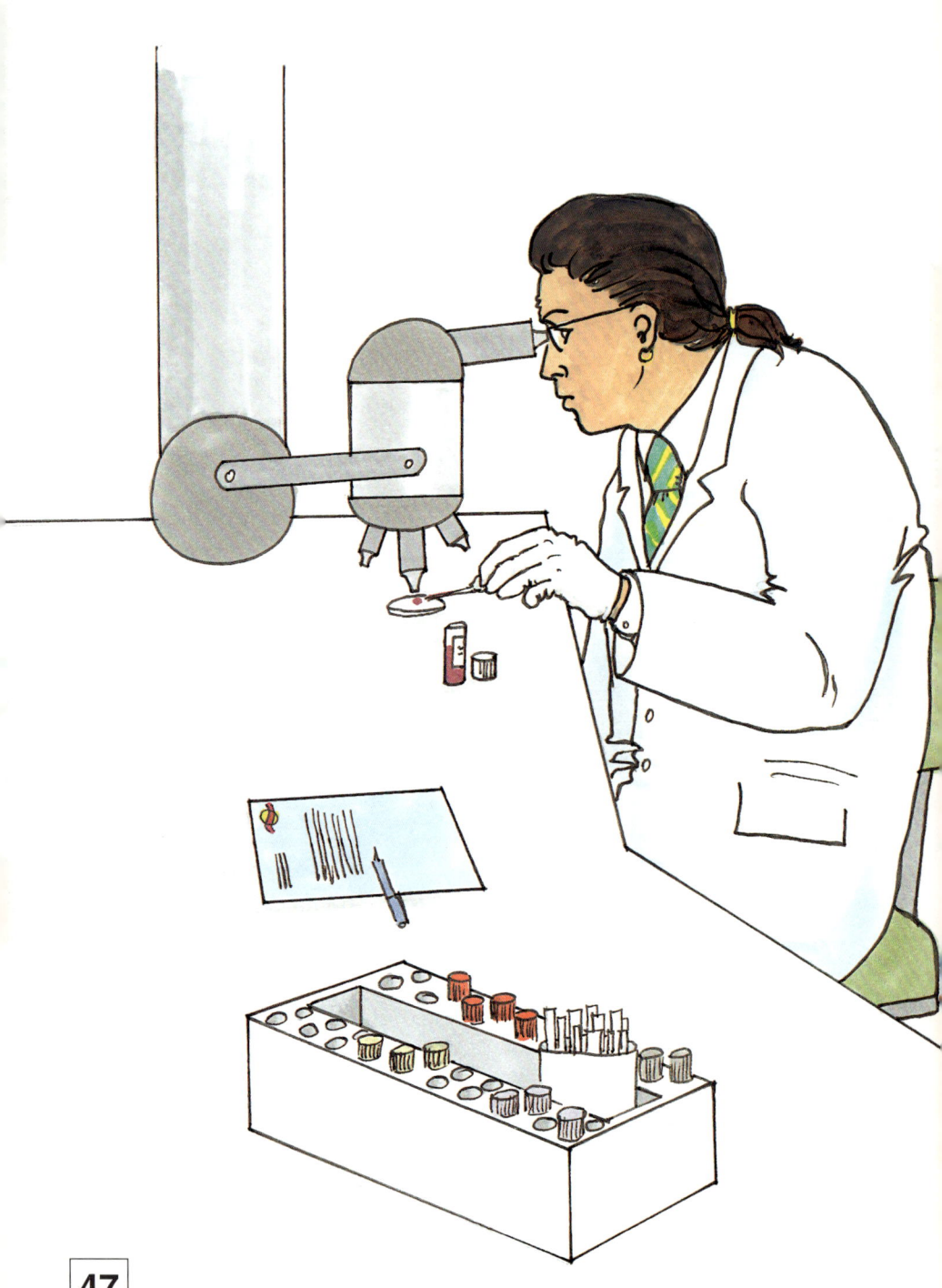

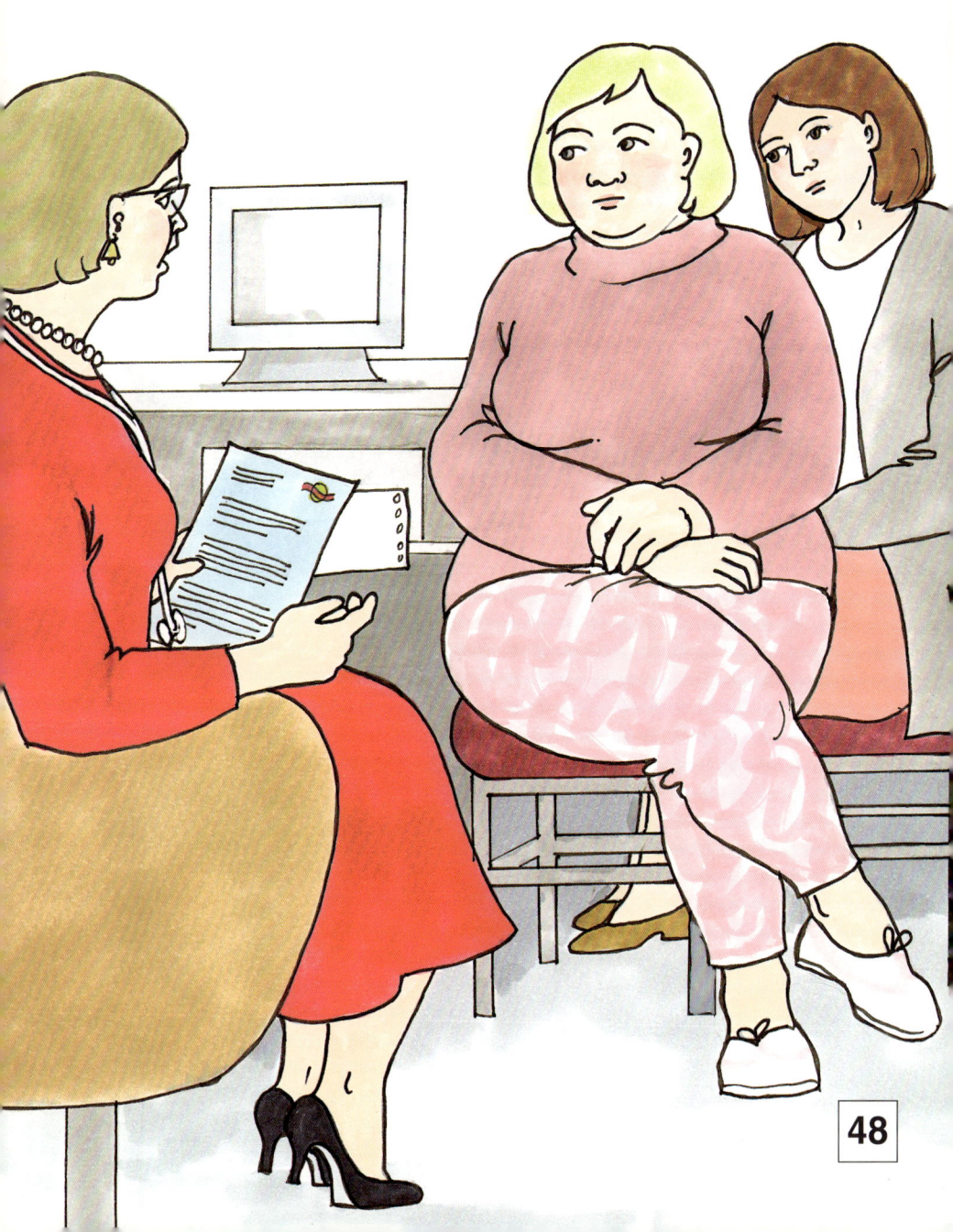
48

'Something to make me better'

The doctor gives Miss Smith a prescription

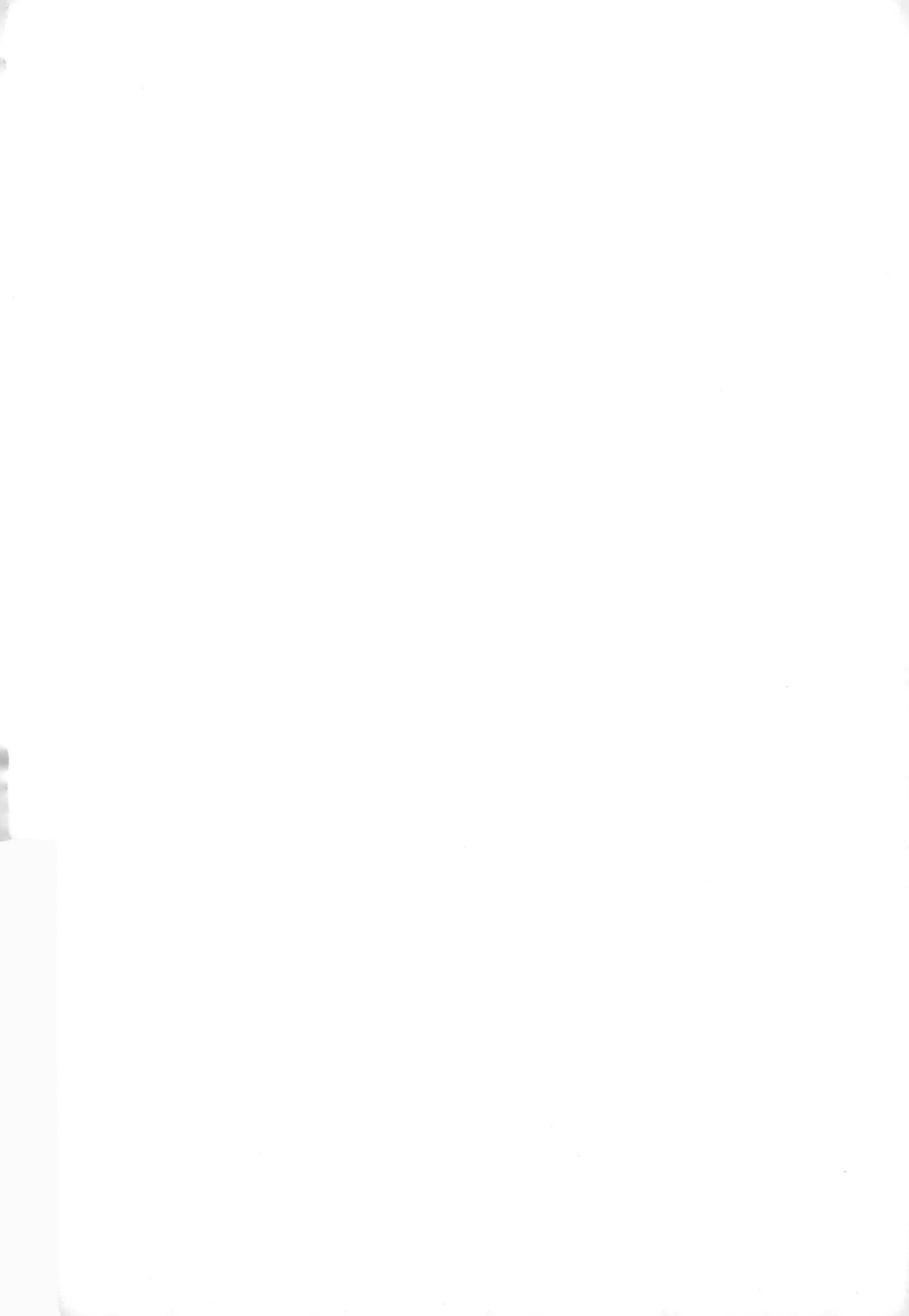

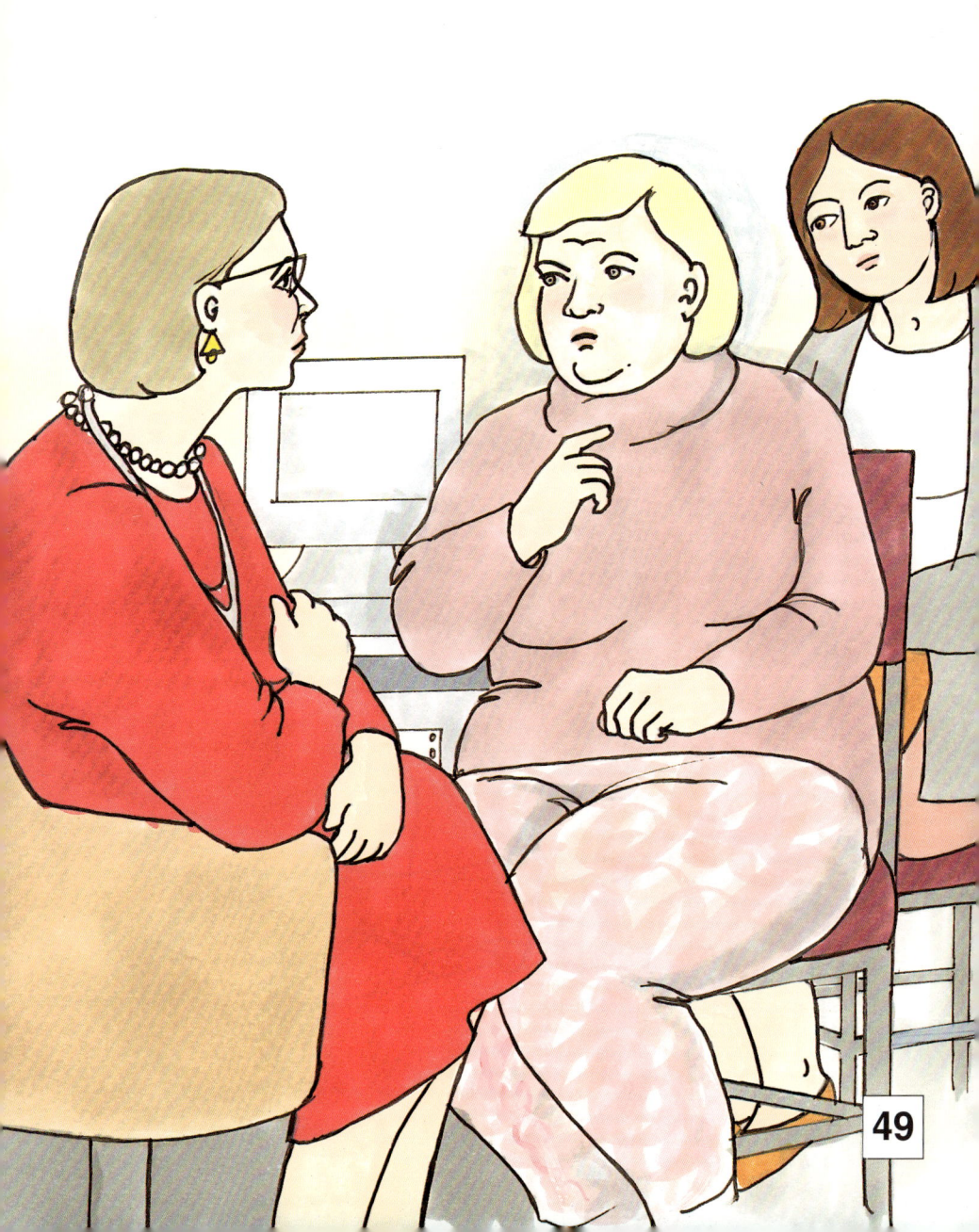

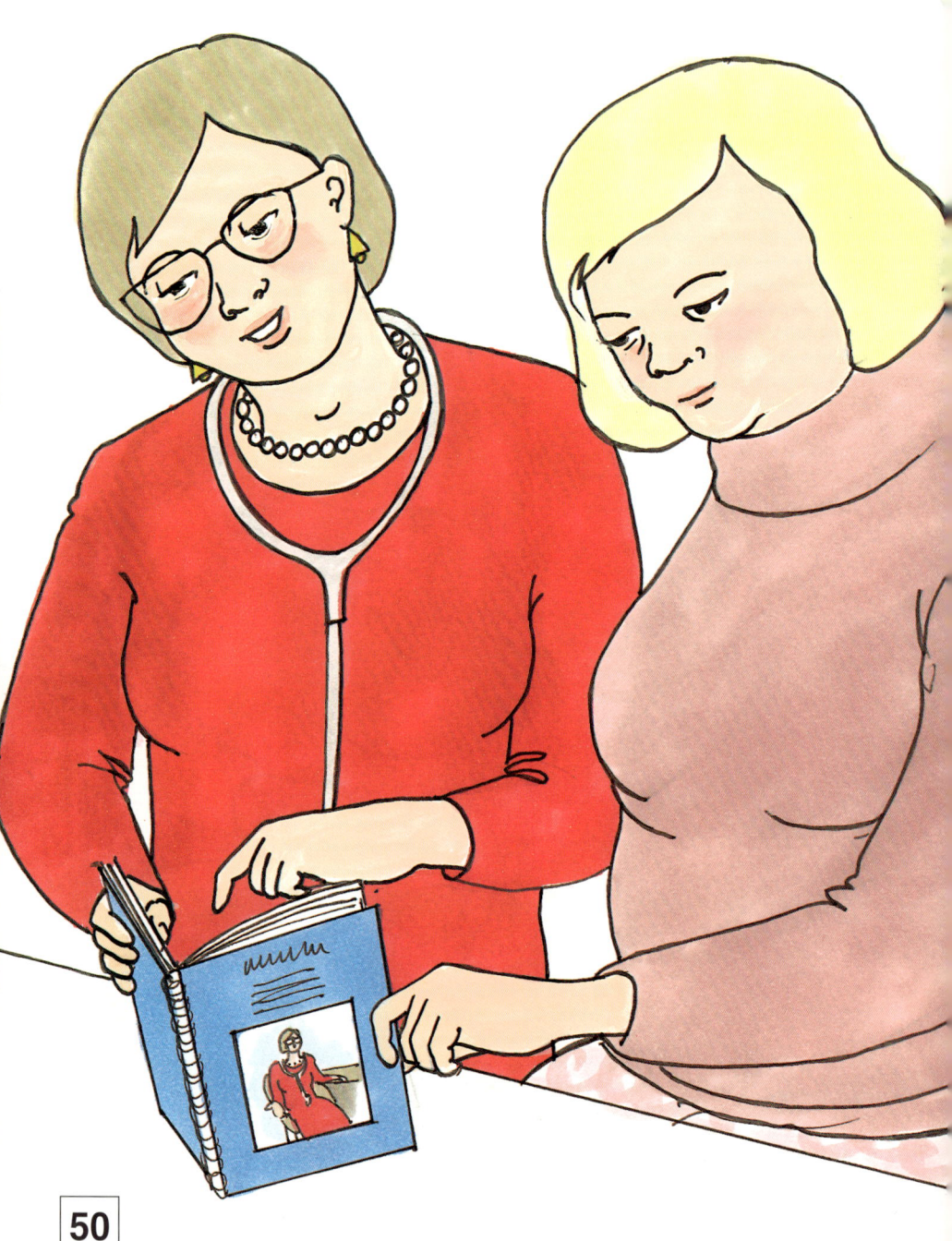

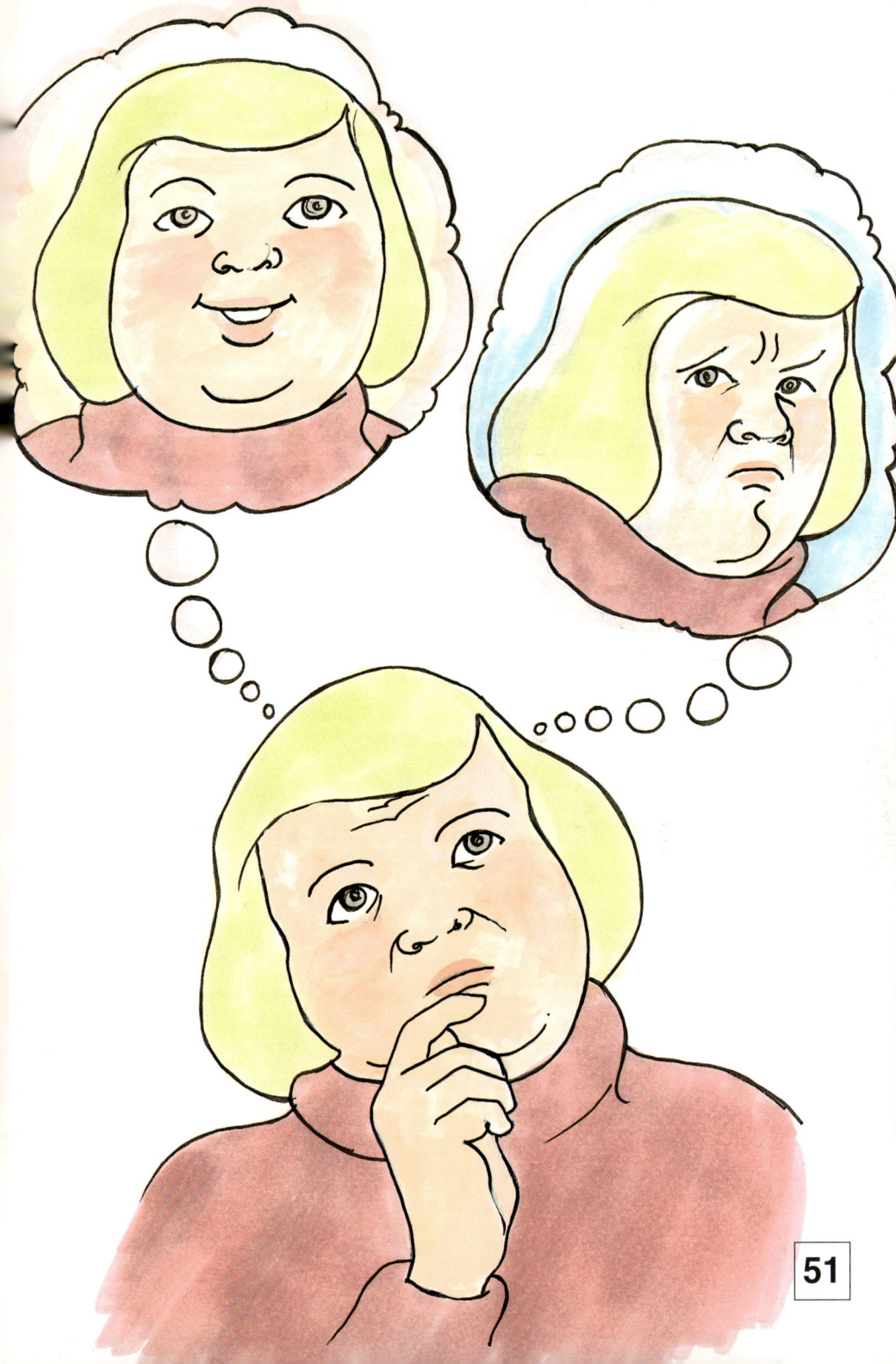

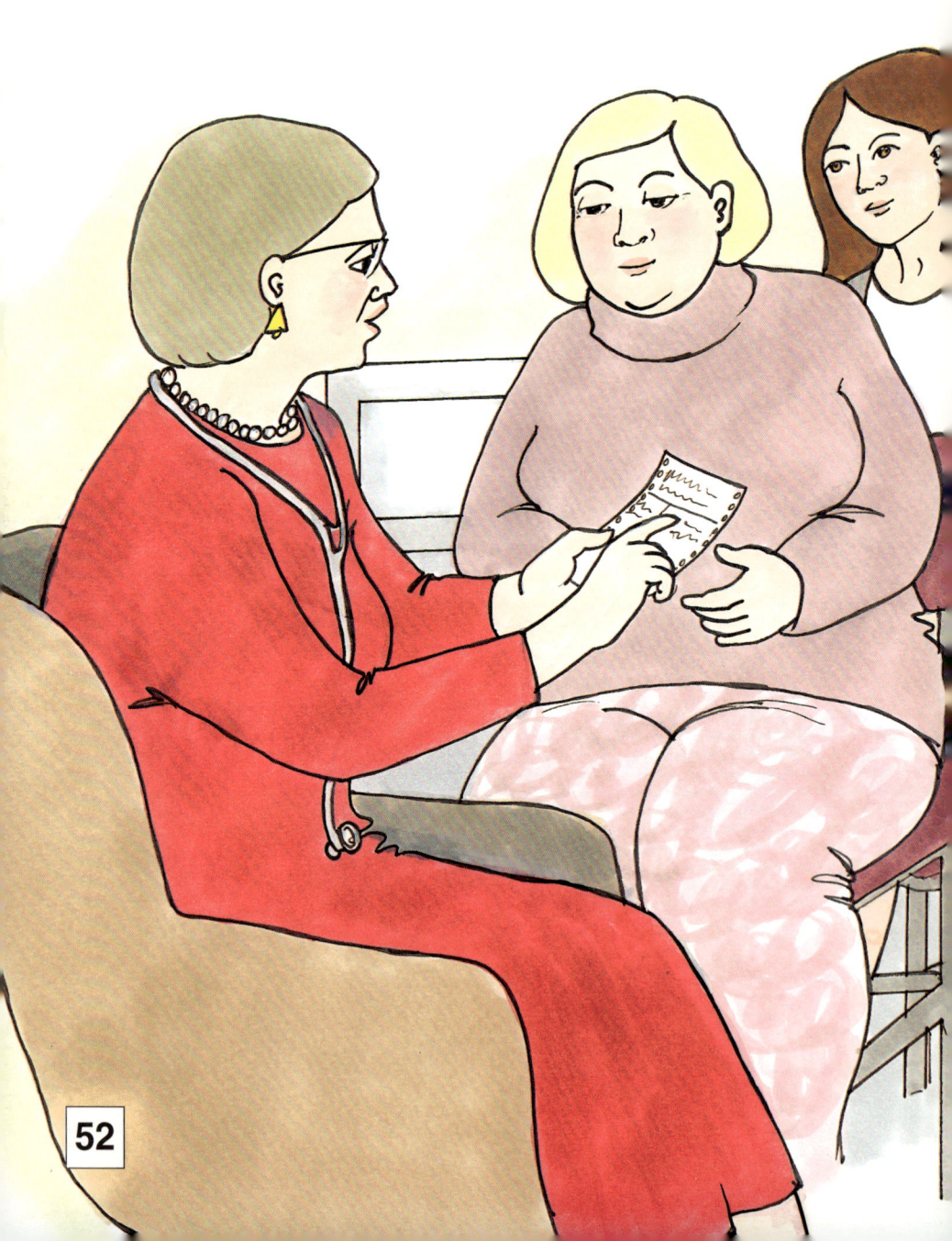

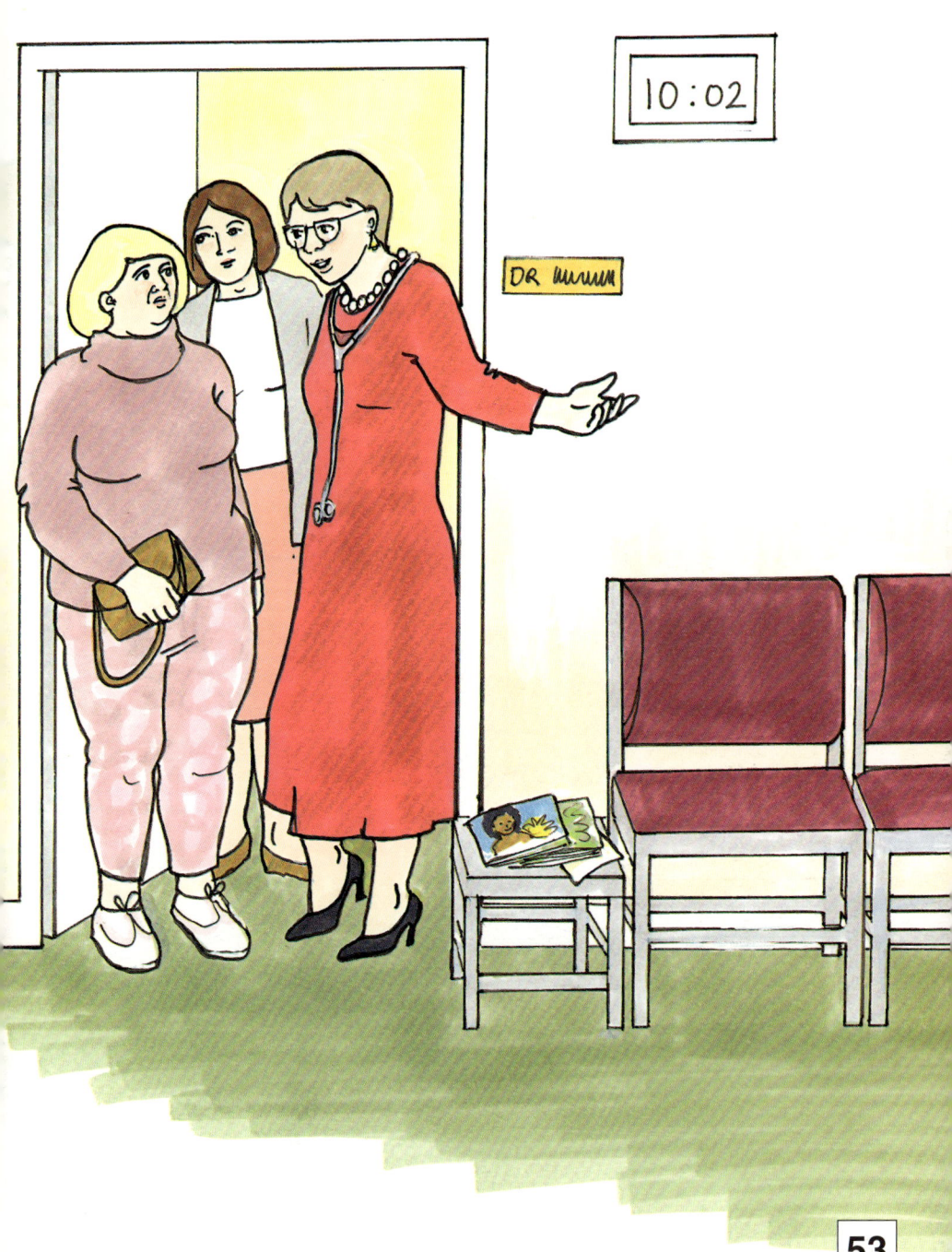

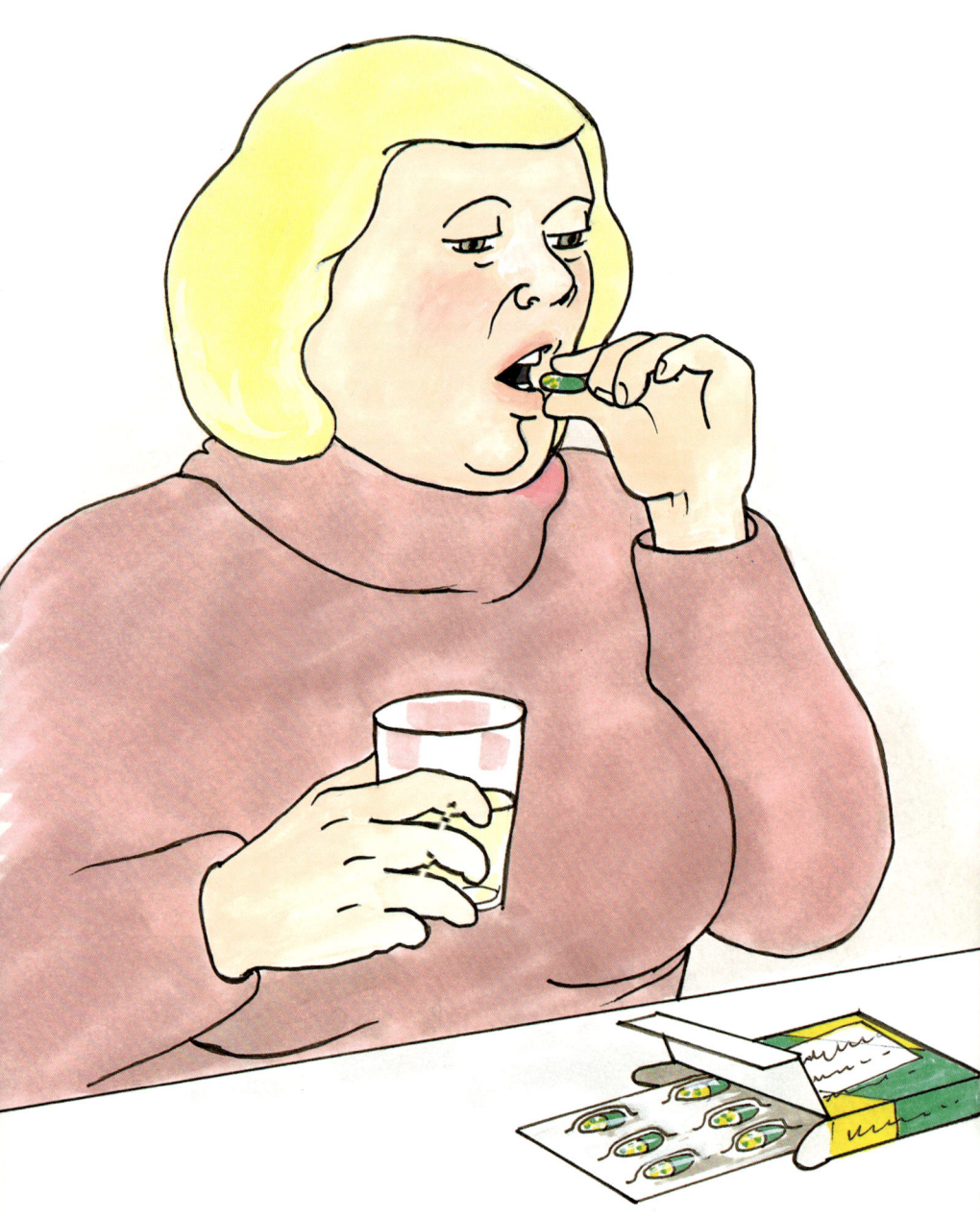

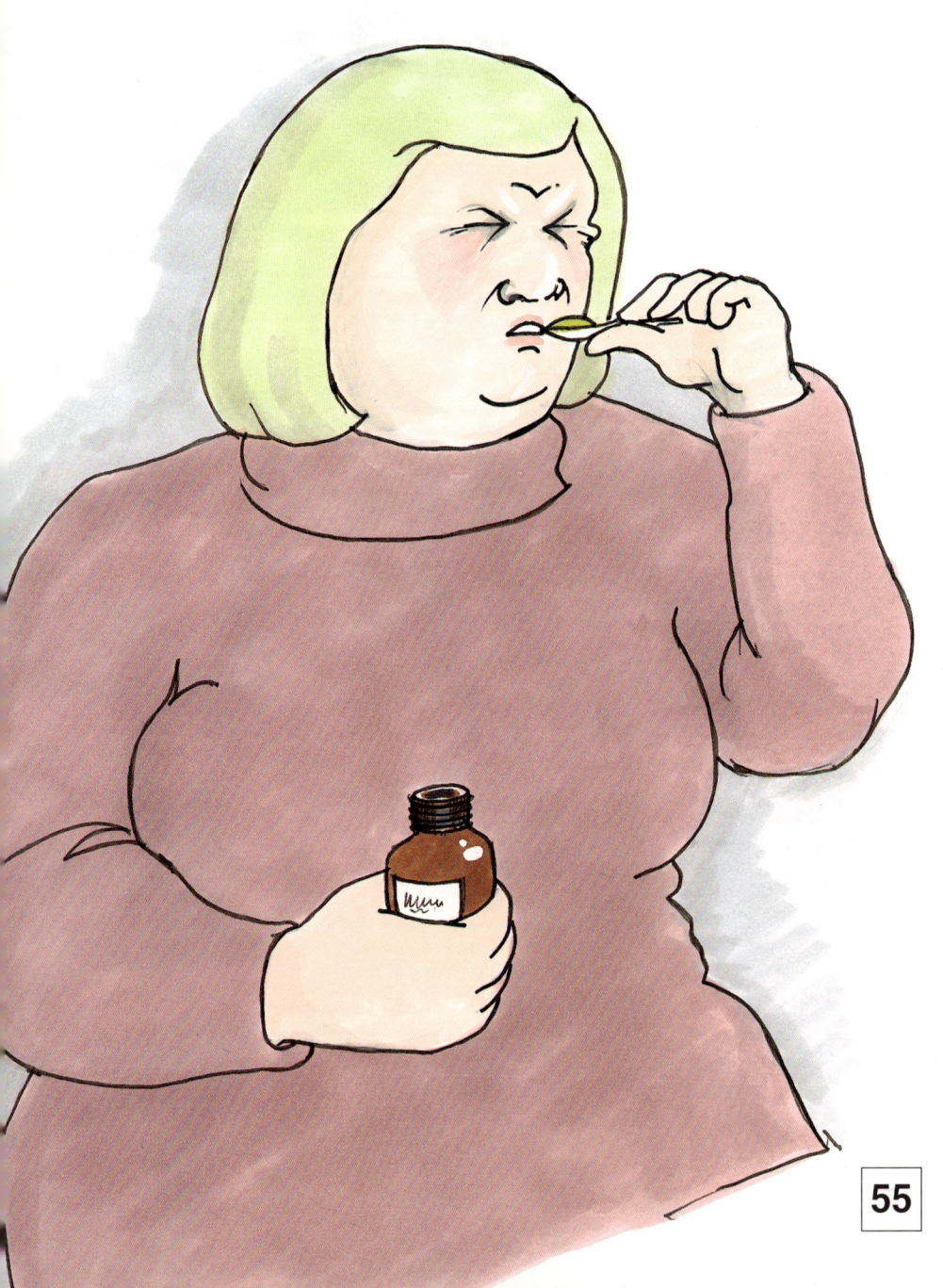

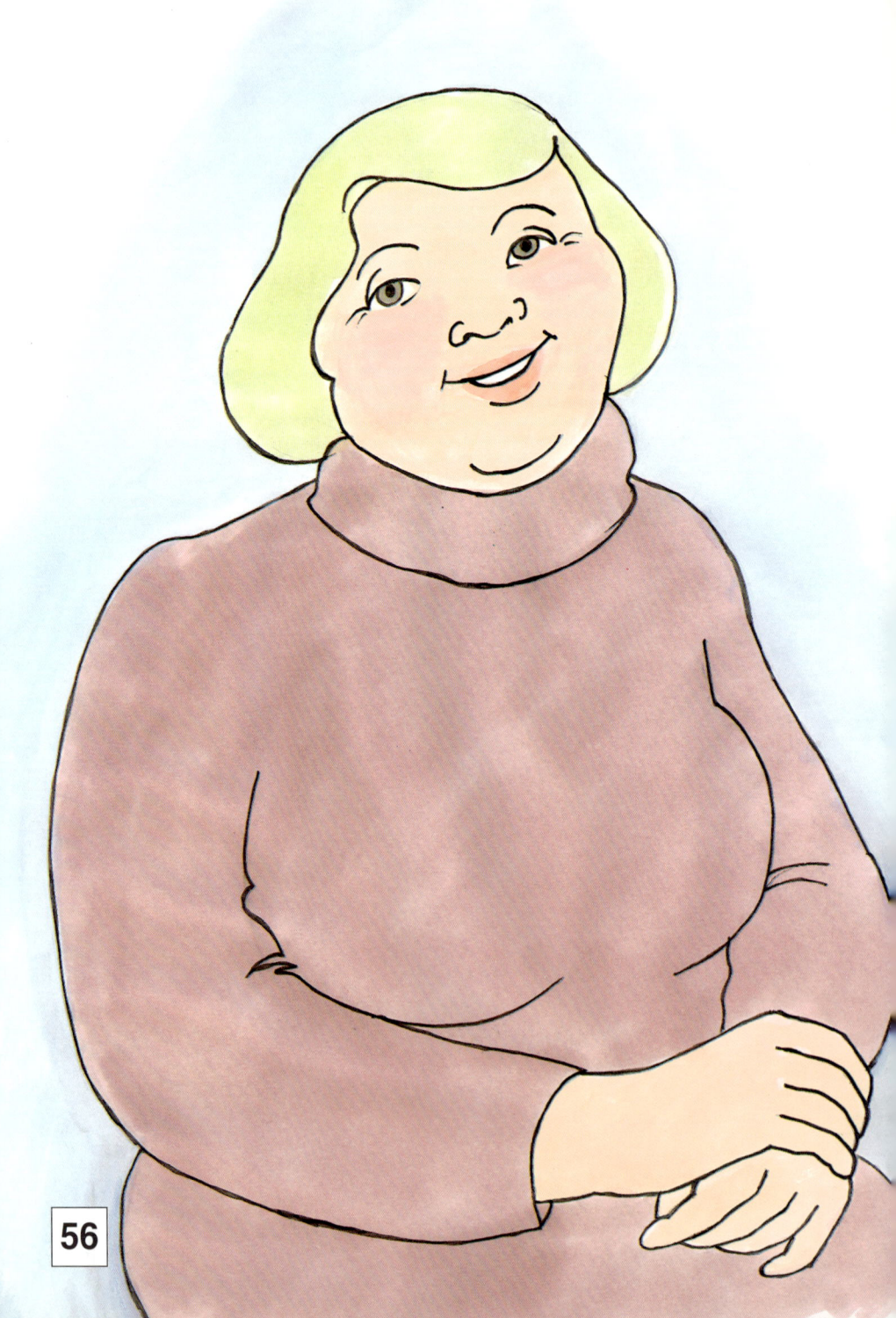

Suggested text for each scenario

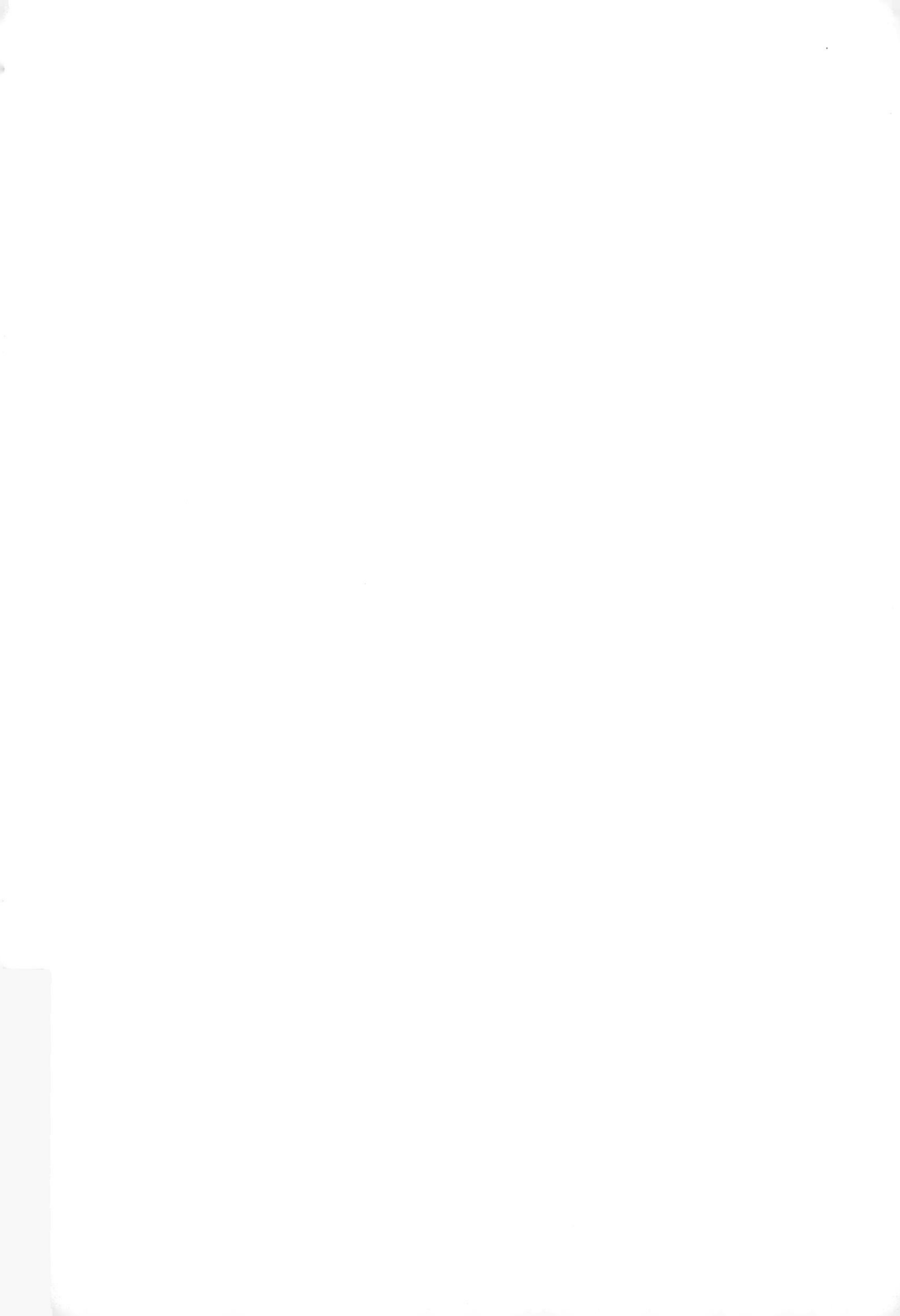

Introduction: Jim Lane and Anne Smith arrive at the Health Centre

1. Jim Lane has an appointment to see the doctor. He goes to the health centre with George, his supporter. Ann Smith also has an appointment. Her friend Joanne goes with her.
2. The notice tells them who works at the centre, and when it is open.
3. "Hello Mr Lane, take a seat. Please wait until the doctor is ready to see you," says the receptionist.
4. The receptionist looks at her book. "Miss Smith? Take a seat over there. Doctor will see you in a minute."
5. Ann and Joanne look at this book. They talk about what happens at the doctor's. Ann is a bit worried about what the doctor might do. She is pleased Joanne has shown her the book. She likes to have time to think about things.
6. "Come in please," says the doctor.
7. The doctor asks what is wrong. "Do you have any pain? Tell me about it," she says

Scenario 1 — Blood pressure

8. Jim tells the doctor how he is feeling. She asks a lot of questions. Jim answers the best he can. Then he says: "This is George, my supporter. Do you want to ask him anything?"

9. The doctor shows Jim what she wants to do. Jim asks her some questions: "Will it hurt?" "Why do you want to do it?" "Will it help me get better?"

10. Jim thinks about what the doctor has said.

    "Do I really want a blood pressure test?"

    Why does the doctor want to do it? What will happen if I don't have the blood pressure test? He has to decide.

    He can say "O.K." to a blood pressure test or "No, thank you".

11. Jim agrees to let the doctor test his blood pressure. The doctor puts a band round his arm.

12. The doctor squeezes a balloon and the band gets tight. She listens to his arm with her stethoscope. Jim's arm feels a bit funny, but she loosens the band again quite quickly.

13. The doctor explains to Jim about his blood pressure. "Is my blood pressure good or bad?" he asks.

14. The doctor answers his questions. "I'm glad that's over," he thinks.

Scenario 2 — The doctor examines Jim Lane's tummy

15. Jim tells the doctor how he is feeling. She asks a lot of questions. Jim answers the best he can. Then he says: "This is George, my supporter. Do you want to ask him anything?"

16. The doctor shows Jim what she wants to do. Jim asks her some questions. "Will it hurt?" "Why do you want to do it?" "Will it help me get better?"

17. Jim thinks about what the doctor has said. "Do I really want to have my tummy examined?"

    "Why does the doctor want to do it?" "What will happen if I don't want to have my tummy examined?" He has to decide.

    He can say "O.K." to his tummy being examined or "No, thank you."

18. Jim agrees to have his tummy examined. The doctor says: "Please go behind the curtains. Please undo your clothes. George can help you if you want. I will come in when you are ready."

19. Jim undoes his trousers. He lies down on the bed. George helps him cover up with a blanket. Jim is embarrassed. George says the doctor needs to see Jim's tummy to find out what is wrong with him.

20. The doctor looks at Jim's tummy. At first she presses gently, but then she pushes harder. She asks Jim to cough. Jim is still embarrassed. He is glad the doctor is looking at his face most of the time. "Tell me if I'm hurting you," she says. She looks at Jim's face to see.

21. Jim does up his clothes. He is glad he brought George with him.

22. The doctor answers his questions. "I'm glad that's over," he thinks.

Scenario 3 — Jim has an injection

23. Jim tells the doctor how he is feeling. She asks a lot of questions. Jim answers the best he can. Then he says: "This is George, my supporter. Do you want to ask him anything?"

24. You need an injection says the doctor. Jim is worried. He asks her some questions. "Will it hurt?" "Will it help me get better?"

25. Jim thinks about what the doctor has said. "Do I really want an injection?"

    "Why does the doctor want to do it?" "What will happen if I don't have the injection?" He has to decide.

    He can say "O.K." to an injection or "No, thank you."

26. The needle looks very long. "Will it hurt a lot?" he asks.

27. The doctor sticks the needle in Jim's arm. "Ouch, that did hurt a bit!" It was not as painful as Jim expected.

28. The doctor puts a plaster on Jim's arm. That wasn't too bad.

29. The doctor answers his questions. "I'm glad that's over," he thinks.

Scenario 4 — Ann Smith has her ears syringed

30. Ann is worried. What is the nurse going to do?
31. "Please come in," says the nurse. Ann and Joanne go into the treatment room.
32. Ann tells the nurse that she can't hear properly.
33. The nurse looks right inside Ann's ear.
34. The nurse explains what she wants to do. Ann asks her some questions. "Will it hurt?" "Why do you want to do it?" "Will it help me get better?" "What will happen if I decide not to let you do it?"
35. Ann thinks about what the nurse said.

    "Do I really want to have my ears washed out?"

    "Why does the nurse want to do that?"

    Ann has to decide.

    She can say "Yes, I will have my ears washed out", or "No, thank you."
36. The nurse wants to wash out Ann's ears with warm water. Ann is a bit frightened. "I hope it doesn't hurt," she thinks.
37. The nurse gives Ann a cup to hold under her ear. She squirts warm water into Ann's ear. It is terribly noisy, but it doesn't hurt.
38. Ann looks in the cup. "Goodness, did all that stuff come out of my ear?" she asks.
39. Ann can hear again! She listens to Joanne's watch ticking. She can hear the birds singing outside in the garden.

Scenario 5 — Ann Smith has a blood test

40. The nurse explains what she wants to do. Ann asks her some questions. "Will it hurt?" "Why do you want to do it?" "Will it help me to get better?" "What will happen if I decide not to let you do it?"

41. Ann thinks about what the nurse has said. "Do I really want a blood test?" Ann has to decide. She can say "Yes" to a blood test or "No, thank you."

42. The nurse puts a tight band round Ann's arm and ask her to keep very still. The nurse has a needle in her hand. Ann is worried. "How much blood will the nurse take?"

43. The nurse tells Ann to look away from the needle. She sticks the needle in Ann's arm. It hurts a little bit.

44. Dark red blood goes into the syringe. The nurse puts the blood into different coloured bottles. She will send Ann's blood to the laboratory.

45. The nurse undoes the band and holds cotton wool over the needle. She pulls the needle out. She tells Ann to press the cotton wool on to her arm.

46. Ann's arm is not bleeding. The nurse sticks a plaster over the place where the needle went in. "You did well," she tells Ann.

47. In the laboratory a man looks at Ann's blood down a microscope.

    He writes down what he sees. He sends a letter to Ann's doctor.

48. Ann goes back to visit the doctor another day.

    The doctor explains the blood test to her. "Is my blood all right?" asks Ann. "Am I getting better? Do I need any treatment?"

Scenario 6 — The doctor gives Ann Smith a prescription

49. Ann talks to the doctor about her problem. The doctor tells Ann what is wrong.
50. The doctor says she needs to take some tablets/medicine.
51. Ann thinks about what the doctor has said.

    Do I really want to take tablets/medicine. Why does the doctor want me to? What will happen if I don't take the tablets/medicine? She has to decide. She can say "O.K. I want the tablets/medicine" or "No, thank you". She asks about the tablets/medicine.

52. "You need to take these tablets/medicine once a day for a week. Please take this prescription to the chemist and they will give you the tablets/medicine." The doctor tells Ann the name of the tablets/medicine and:

    - what the tablets are for
    - what time of day to take them
    - how to take them; how long to go on taking them
    - what to do if she misses a dose
    - whether she can drink alcohol while she is taking the tablets
    - whether she can use machinery while she is taking the tablets
    - what odd things (side effects) the tablets may do
    - and who to ask if she is worried.

53. "Goodbye. I hope you feel better soon."
54. Ann takes the tablets (before lunch) with a glass of water.
55. Ann swallows a spoonful of the medicine (every evening).
56. Ann feels much better now.

Guide for supporters

How to Use this Book

A Guide for Supporters/Informants

Supporters are the people whom individuals trust and feel safe with when going to the doctor. They can be parents or other family members, friends or advocates or staff members.

This book is designed to support people with a learning disability when visiting their doctor. It can be used at the GP's surgery to explain some common events such as an ear examination or measurement of blood pressure. It will be useful to look at it before going to the doctor to give information and explore feelings. The book is also designed to be used by staff as part of their health promotion and education work in different settings.

The book pictures events as commonplace as arriving at a reception desk and sitting in a waiting room to some less pleasant experiences that may involve embarrassment and some pain. The pictures are intended to assist understanding and aid communication. Some ideas in the story are prompts, for example about consent and understanding and about medicines.

At the Doctor's Surgery

Copies of the book should be made available to people with a learning disability and their supporters who have come to see their GP. The book follows two people Jim Lane and Ann Smith arriving at the surgery. The different sections of the book explain in picture form some of the most common experiences that either Jim or Ann may have. There are six 'stories' or scenarios in this book; having blood pressure taken, examination of the abdomen, an injection in the arm, ear examination and syringing, taking a blood sample, and how medicine is prescribed.

It is usually advisable that the pictures are looked at in order and only the sequence most relevant to that visit is used. In addition to the scenarios there are sections covering consent to treatment and investigations. These should be referred to after each scenario. You may need to set aside time to allow the person to follow the picture sequence at their own pace.

Before Going to the Doctor

This book can also be used to help explain some of the things that may happen in advance. By following the appropriate picture sequence the individual can be prepared for planned events such as a blood test or ear syringe. At the end of the pictures are descriptive story captions which you can use. The pictures can be used to check the person's understanding by discussing how Jim or Ann might be feeling at different stages of their visit. You may also want to check that the person understands who the different people in the picture are and what Jim and Ann are doing, e.g. talking to the receptionist, sitting in the waiting room, seeing the doctor etc.

It is important that only the sections that most concern the individual are referred to as part of preparation.

Health Education and Promotion

Parts of the book may be helpful when planning health education work. Group work can be used to share experiences portrayed in the picture sequences and peer support can help reduce anxiety. Groups can role play how to organise going to the doctor, talking to their supporters and making an appointment, as well as attending the surgery or health centre itself.

A leaflet is available from the publisher which gives more information about the Books Beyond Words series and how to use these books with people with learning disabilities.

Medical words explained

Medical Words Explained

Blood Pressure: the force that pushes or pumps blood around the body is called blood pressure. A doctor or nurse can tell you what your blood pressure is by listening to it going through your arm. This does not hurt. Most people have 'normal' blood pressure, but sometimes it can be too 'high' and the doctor can help get it back to normal.

Ear Syringe: usually a metal tube that a nurse uses to wash wax out of the ear. The tube is filled with warm water and gently put a little way into the ear. The water and wax comes out of the ear by itself and is collected in a bowl. It doesn't hurt but it may make you feel dizzy.

Injection: an injection is a way of giving medicine into your body through a needle. Injections are usually given in the arm or the bottom. They do hurt a little bit.

Examination: this means looking to see how you are. The doctor may look at your ears by shining a light or listen to your chest as you breath in and out. It can also mean looking where you feel pain, your arm or leg or tummy, and you may have to take some clothes off for the doctor to see. The doctor may also want to touch the part of your body that he/she is looking at.

Blood test: the doctor may want to take a little bit of blood to see if it's O.K. Maybe the doctor needs to know if the medicine you're taking is working properly, or maybe to see if you've got something wrong with your blood. To do this the doctor or nurse will use a needle and some special bottles. The needle pricks your arm and the blood goes in the bottle. This does hurt a little bit and you may want to look away.

Prescription: the doctor writes down any medicine, tablets or capsules you need to take on a piece of paper called a prescription. When you take this to the chemist you will be given the medicine that the doctor has written down. Some doctors write the prescription with a pen and others with their computer.

Receptionist: this is the person you see first before seeing your doctor. Sometimes they sit behind a counter. You can make an appointment to see your doctor with the receptionist. You will be told when the doctor can see you. When you go to the surgery tell the receptionist who you are. Also tell her who you've come to see before sitting in the waiting area.

Treatment Room: this is the room where the nurse works. The nurse helps the doctor in different ways, like washing out the wax from people's ears or taking their blood pressure or weighing people to see how heavy they are.

Health Centre/Surgery: this is the building where your doctor works. Most health centres and surgeries have a receptionist and a waiting area. Nurses also work at the health centre and some health centres have chiropodists who look after feet and dentists who look after teeth.

Laboratory: the blood that has been taken out of your arm is sent to a place called a laboratory to be looked at. The laboratory then tells the doctor how your blood is by sending a letter to the health centre.

A Guide for GPs and the Primary Care Team

(includes definition of learning disability)

A Guide for General Practitioners and the Primary Care Team

This book is designed to help your patients with a learning disability use their GPs more effectively by explaining six common events; having blood pressure taken, examination of the abdomen, an injection in the arm, how medicine is prescribed, ear examination and syringing and taking a blood sample. This is a pictorial communication tool, and its use is not confined to people who do not speak. Many people with a learning disability find associating a picture with the information that you give very helpful.

The pictures are in sequence and can either be used before attending the surgery by way of preparation or while at the surgery. This will enable the patient to ask appropriate questions, and help you to obtain truly informed consent. This advice on how to use the book is followed by a list of suggested health checks for people with learning disability in general, and specifically Down's Syndrome, one of the commonest causes of learning disability.

Definition of Learning Disability

People said to have a 'learning disability' have a reduced ability to understand new or complex information and may not be able to cope independently. Some people are known to have a learning disability from birth, such as people with Down's Syndrome, but for all of these patients their condition will have started before adulthood and have a lasting impact on development. (Based on definition in Health of the Nation, 1995.)

Having a learning disability does not mean that the person will never understand the advice or treatment you give. Some will not need this book to assist their understanding and will have good communication skills. A very few will find all information bewildering and will not have the comprehension to follow a sequence of pictures. Sometimes one or two carefully chosen pictures will be enough to explain what is going to happen. Many people with learning disabilities need time and patient support to understand information, whether presented in simplified language or non verbally.

Supporter/Informant: Some people with learning disability will come to the surgery with a family member, advocate or staff member whose role it is to support their attendance and assist communication. The patient often relies on the supporter to help describe symptoms and other information, and may need time and encouragement to participate in the doctor-patient relationship rather than depending too much on the informant speaking for them.

Augmentative communication: this book is an example of a different way in which your verbal communication with the patient can be augmented, in this case pictorially. Many people with a learning disability use signs or symbols to augment or substitute for spoken language (e.g. Makaton or Bliss). The person who accompanies the patient should be skilled in whatever communication system the patient uses.

Consent

This book emphasises the issue of consent and provides pictures that may help to clarify the choices open to the patient.

Doctors are often worried about consent in people with learning disabilities. The advice that follows is closely based on the relevant section of Assessment of Mental Capacity 1995 BMA/Law Society. The assessment of an adult patient's capacity to make a decision about his or her own medical treatment is a matter for clinical judgement, guided by professional practice and subject to legal requirements. It is the personal responsibility of any doctor proposing to treat a patient to judge whether that person has the capacity to give a valid consent.

To demonstrate capacity individuals should be able to:
- understand in simple language what the treatment is, its purpose and nature and why it is being proposed
- understand its principal benefits, risks and alternatives
- retain the information for long enough to make an effective decision
- make a free choice (i.e. free from pressure).

Many people with learning disability will be able to give valid consent if the explanation is simple and repeated. Augmented communication may be useful for some people. The capacity to write is not important, a witnessed mark or thumb print will suffice.

A few people with learning disabilities will lack the capacity to consent. In this situation the doctor must proceed in good faith when such treatment is in the patient's best interests, consistent with the doctor's duty of care. Acting in good faith will usually involve discussing the case with relatives or other significant persons. However, the present state of English Law means that no one can give legally valid consent to medical treatment on behalf of another adult. The law on competency and consent may change in the near future and practitioners need to make themselves aware of the current law on consent.

Suggested health surveillance and health promotion for patients with learning disability

- Inclusion in population based screening/health promotion

In addition

- Establish primary cause of learning disability if possible, since it may have further health implications
- Vision
- Hearing
- Mobility and posture — check for spinal deformity and evaluate need for therapy and or equipment
- Sleep — problems are common
- Weight — changes may indicate poor diet, lack of exercise, thyroid disorder or depression, all relatively common missed diagnoses in this group
- Immunisation — especially important where people still live in large institutions — Hepatitis A & B and influenza
- Drugs — avoid long term unmonitored use of drugs especially neuroleptics and polypharmacy
- Epilepsy — regular review of seizures, medication and side effects
- Emotional distress and behavioural disturbance:

    (1) may be a response to abuse, bereavement or other life changes. May need referral for behavioural, psychotherapeutic or drug treatment

    (2) may be a response to a physical illness or symptom including pain

- Carer's health and plans for the future
- Care — signs of poor care, e.g. halitosis, blepharitis, pressure sores may indicate a deterioration in the person's function or that carers are not coping

Suggestion: Photocopy this page and include in the notes of each patient with a learning disability.

Routine Checks in Down's Syndrome

People with Down's Syndrome are at increased risk for a number of medical conditions.

To be done once:
- immunisation — hepatitis A & B
- congenital heart disease (CHD)

To be done regularly:
- T4 (increased risk of thyroid disease)
- vision check (especially for cataracts)
- hearing check
- influenza prophylaxis
- check for pulmonary hypertension (if CHD present)
- haematology (for anaemia and leukaemia)

To be done when necessary:
- dental prophylaxis if patient has CHD
- adenoidectomy
- grommets
- lateral neck x-ray if signs of cord compression appear
- treat febrile illnesses promptly with antipyretics

Suggestion: Photocopy this page and include in the notes of each patient with Down's Syndrome.

Useful Resources

Services

Community Teams for People with a Learning Disability [CTPLD]: multidisciplinary health teams that support clients, their families and services, by assessment of their health needs and a range of clinical interventions. The composition of CTPLDs varies, but will usually include psychiatry, psychology and nursing with a range of therapeutic specialists such as speech and language therapy, occupational therapy and physiotherapy. Referral to the local CTPLD is encouraged for both developmental and therapeutic work. Some teams are joint health and social work teams and have a social care management role as well.

Social Service Departments: Social Service departments manage and purchase social care, for example, housing and day services for people with learning disabilities.

Written material

BMA/Law Society (1995). Assessment of Mental Capacity: Guidance for Doctors and Lawyers. London: British Medical Association.

Contact a Family Directory, 170 Tottenham Court Road, London W1P OHA. Tel No: 0171 383 3555

Department of Health (1995). The Health of the Nation: A strategy for people with learning disabilities. London: Department of Health.

Health Education Authority (1995). Health Related Resources for People with Learning Disabilities. London: Health Education Authority.

Health Related Resources for People with Learning Disabilities database, The Health Promotion Information Centre, Health Education Authority, Hamilton House, Mabledon Place, London WC1 9TX.

Royal College of General Practitioners (1990). Primary Care for People with a Mental Handicap. Occasional Paper 47. London: Royal College of General Practitioners

Thompson D. (1993), Learning Disabilities: The fundamental facts. London: The Mental Health Foundation.

Organisations

Useful contact numbers:

Fragile X Society (parent contact)
53 Winchelsea Lane,
Hastings,
East Sussex
TN35 4LG　　　　　　　　　　　　　　　01424 813147

MENCAP
123 Golden Lane,
London
EC1Y 0RT　　　　　　　　　　　　　　0171 454 0454

National Autistic Society
276 Willesden Lane,
London
NW2 5RB　　　　　　　　　　　　　　0181 451 1114

National Society for Epilepsy
Chalfont St Peter,
Buckinghamshire
SL9 0RJ　　　　　　　　　　　　　　　01494 873991

People First,
207-215 Kings Cross Road,
London
WC1X 9DB　　　　　　　　　　　　　　0171 713 6400
(a self advocacy organisation run by people with learning disability)

SCOPE
12 Park Crescent,
London
W1N 4EQ　　　　　　　　　　　　　　0171 636 5020